Y0-BZT-509

What people are saying about

Resetting Our Future:

Long Haul COVID: A Survivor's Guide

Long Haul COVID: A Survivor's Guide: Transform Your Pain & Find Your Way Forward by Dr. Joseph Trunzo and Julie Luongo is a much welcomed and needed book that not only addresses the severe emotional impact of COVID-19 but more importantly, offers a unique method for living a fruitful life once again.

This book is appropriate for both the public and professionals. Dr. Trunzo is an expert in Acceptance and Commitment Therapy (ACT), an evidenced-based contextual behavioral approach aimed at increasing psychological flexibility in order to address a number of emotional and behavioral-health issues. As he did in his previous book *Living Beyond Lyme*, Dr. Trunzo again lays a creative foundation for applying the processes of ACT to Long Haul COVID sufferers.

This is not your everyday run-in-the mill self-help book. It is well constructed, offering numerous experiential exercises, metaphors, and mindfulness meditations. Throughout the book Dr. Trunzo starts with an overview of each ACT process, then Julie Luongo illustrates how these processes are applied via her real-life experience. A running theme that restores the reader's hope in regaining emotional wellness is a constant emphasis on achieving psychological flexibility; a perspective that shows how to live a value-chosen life even in the face of hardship. As Dr. Trunzo states very clearly, this comes in the way of practicing the six ACT processes.

This book is a special gift to humanity given the immense amount of loss, isolation, and sadness that we all have experienced. Dr. Trunzo eloquently captures the power in all of us to transform desperate conditions into positivity, and by doing so, provides a beacon of hope for living a fulfilling life after the pandemic.

Andrew J. D'Amico, PhD, Psychologist and Past President of the Pennsylvania Chapter of the Association of Contextual & Behavioral Sciences

Dr Trunzo and Ms. Luongo present here a work of great importance during this unprecedented time in human history... specifically OUR personal history. The COVID pandemic has claimed more lives worldwide in the shortest time since its outbreak compared to any other pandemic in history. They inject a voice of authority and calm, guiding us on how to cope with losses, financial and relations. They walk us through each stage of our human and public challenges of the time and lead us with a steady hand in applying the concepts of ACT therapy. As a psychiatrist I find this immensely helpful in helping my own patients make sense of and cope in these most challenging of times.

Mo Dattu, M.D., Founder of Psychiatric Practice, LLC

This book is an invaluable and easily accessible guide to helping individuals cope and thrive with the challenging impact of Long Haul COVID. It is also useful to any of us dealing with the impact of living through a pandemic and to individuals who have other health conditions. Dr. Trunzo presents a clear description of the scientifically supported approach called Acceptance and Commitment Therapy (ACT), including easy to follow instructions, metaphors and exercises to help apply this approach to coping with Long Haul COVID and the impact this condition can have on functioning and quality of life. These concepts are then brought to life in each chapter through Julie Luongo's personal accounts with Long Haul COVID and her tips to readers based on her experience with applying ACT to help her cope and function more fully in life. This book is easy to read and implement and can have the powerful effect of allowing readers to pursue a fulfilling life even in the face of Long Haul COVID. As a psychologist, I have experienced the impact of ACT with clients, including those suffering from medical conditions. I highly recommend this impactful book that is truly a gift to patients with Long Haul COVID and the family and friends who support them, as well as to other clinicians, including therapists and medical providers who treat patients with this condition. In fact, I recommend this book to anyone who has been dealing with the various stressors related to the pandemic and also to individuals and caregivers dealing with other health conditions.

Dina Harth, PhD, Licensed Psychologist, Vice-President, Pennsylvania Chapter of the Association of Contextual & Behavioral Science

Joe Trunzo and Julie Luongo have packed so much helpful guidance into a concise and easily accessible volume. They deliver on the promise of their sub-title to "Transform Your Pain and Find Your Way Forward," so that we can make meaning and purpose amid our Covid challenges and craft a life that keeps us connected to the things that deeply matter to us. Joseph's writing is uncommonly clear, direct, and simple to put into practice, while Julie's personal examples give life and context, so we can imagine how to apply their approach in our own unique pandemic circumstances.

John Armando, LCSW

Resetting Our Future

Long Haul COVID: A Survivor's Guide

Transform Your Pain and Find Your Way Forward

Previous Titles

Living Beyond Lyme: Reclaim Your Life from Lyme Disease and Chronic Illness
By Joseph J. Trunzo, PhD
ISBN: 1785350412

The Hard Way
By Julie Luongo
ISBN: 978-0765316677

RESETTING OUR FUTURE

Long Haul COVID: A Survivor's Guide

Transform Your Pain and Find Your Way Forward

Joseph J. Trunzo, Julie Luongo

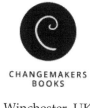

CHANGEMAKERS
BOOKS

Winchester, UK
Washington, USA

JOHN HUNT PUBLISHING

First published by Changemakers Books, 2021
Changemakers Books is an imprint of John Hunt Publishing Ltd., No. 3 East Street,
Alresford, Hampshire SO24 9EE, UK
office@jhpbooks.com
www.johnhuntpublishing.com
www.changemakers-books.com

For distributor details and how to order please visit the 'Ordering' section on our website.

Text copyright: Joseph J. Trunzo and Julie Luongo 2021

ISBN: 978 1 78904 814 8
978 1 78904 815 5 (ebook)
Library of Congress Control Number: 2021937364

All rights reserved. Except for brief quotations in critical articles or reviews, no part of this
book may be reproduced in any manner without prior written permission from the publishers.

The rights of Joseph J. Trunzo and Julie Luongo as authors have been asserted in accordance
with the Copyright, Designs and Patents Act 1988.

A CIP catalogue record for this book is available from the British Library.

Design: Stuart Davies

UK: Printed and bound by CPI Group (UK) Ltd, Croydon, CR0 4YY
Printed in North America by CPI GPS partners

We operate a distinctive and ethical publishing philosophy in
all areas of our business, from our global network of authors to
production and worldwide distribution.

Contents

The *Resetting Our Future* Series

At this critical moment of history, with a pandemic raging, we have the rare opportunity for a Great Reset – to choose a different future. This series provides a platform for pragmatic thought leaders to share their vision for change based on their deep expertise. For communities and nations struggling to cope with the crisis, these books will provide a burst of hope and energy to help us take the first difficult steps towards a better future.

– Tim Ward, publisher, Changemakers Books

What if Solving the Climate Crisis Is Simple?
Tom Bowman, President of Bowman Change, Inc., and writing-team lead for the U.S. ACE National Strategic Planning Framework

Zero Waste Living, the 80/20 Way
The Busy Person's Guide to a Lighter Footprint
Stephanie Miller, Founder of Zero Waste in DC, and former Director, IFC Climate Business Department

A Chicken Can't Lay a Duck Egg
How COVID-19 Can Solve the Climate Crisis
Graeme Maxton, (former Secretary-General of the Club of Rome), and Bernice Maxton-Lee (former Director, Jane Goodall Institute)

A Global Playbook for the Next Pandemic
Anne Kabagambe, former World Bank Executive Director

Power Switch
How We Can Reverse Extreme Inequality
Paul O'Brien, Executive Director, Amnesty International USA

Impact ED
How Community College Entrepreneurship Creates Equity and Prosperity
Rebecca Corbin (President & CEO, National Association of Community College Entrepreneurship), Andrew Gold and Mary Beth Kerly (both business faculty, Hillsborough Community College)

Empowering Climate Action in the United States
Tom Bowman (President of Bowman Change, Inc.) and Deb Morrison (Learning Scientist, University of Washington)

Learning from Tomorrow
Using Strategic Foresight to Prepare for the Next Big Disruption
Bart Édes, former North American Representative, Asian Development Bank

Cut Super Climate Pollutants, Now!
The Ozone Treaty's Urgent Lessons for Speeding Up Climate Action
Alan Miller (former World Bank representative for global climate negotiations), Durwood Zaelke (President and founder, the Institute for Governance & Sustainable Development) and Stephen O. Andersen (former Director of Strategic Climate Projects at the Environmental Protection Agency)

Resetting Our Future: Long Haul COVID: A Survivor's Guide
Transform Your Pain & Find Your Way Forward
Dr. Joseph J. Trunzo (Professor of Psychology and Department Chair at Bryant University), and Julie Luongo (author of *The Hard Way*).

SMART Futures for a Flourishing World
A Paradigm Shift for Achieving the Sustainable Development Goals
Dr. Claire Nelson, Chief Visionary Officer and Lead Futurist,
The Futures Forum

Lead Different
*Designing a Post-COVID Paradigm for Thriving at Work
and at Home*
Monica Brand, Lisa Neuberger & Wendy Teleki

Resetting the Table
Nicole Civita (Vice President of Strategic Initiatives at Sterling
College, Ethics Transformation in Food Systems) and
Michelle Auerbach

Reconstructing Blackness
Rev. Charles Howard, Chaplin, University of Pennsylvania

www.ResettingOurFuture.com

Dedicated to all who have suffered and survived COVID-19.
You are not alone.

Foreword

by Thomas Lovejoy

The pandemic has changed our world. Lives have been lost. Livelihoods as well. Far too many face urgent problems of health and economic security, but almost all of us are reinventing our lives in one way or another. Meeting the immediate needs of the less fortunate is obviously a priority, and a big one. But beyond those compassionate imperatives, there is also tremendous opportunity for what some people are calling a "Great Reset." This series of books, Resetting Our Future, is designed to provide pragmatic visionary ideas and stimulate a fundamental rethink of the future of humanity, nature and the economy.

I find myself thinking about my parents, who had lived through the Second World War and the Great Depression, and am still impressed by the sense of frugality they had attained. When packages arrived in the mail, my father would save the paper and string; he did it so systematically I don't recall our ever having to buy string. Our diets were more careful: whether it could be afforded or not, beef was restricted to once a week. When aluminum foil—the great boon to the kitchen—appeared, we used and washed it repeatedly until it fell apart. Bottles, whether Coca-Cola or milk, were recycled.

Waste was consciously avoided. My childhood task was to put out the trash; what goes out of my backdoor today is an unnecessary multiple of that. At least some of it now goes to recycling but a lot more should surely be possible.

There was also a widespread sense of service to a larger community. Military service was required of all. But there was also the Civilian Conservation Corps, which had provided jobs and repaired the ecological destruction that had generated the Dust Bowl. The Kennedy administration introduced the Peace

Corps and the President's phrase "Ask not what your country can do for you but what you can do for your country" still resonates in our minds.

There had been antecedents, but in the 1970s there was a global awakening about a growing environmental crisis. In 1972, The United Nations held its first conference on the environment at Stockholm. Most of the modern US institutions and laws about environment were established under moderate Republican administrations (Nixon and Ford). Environment was seen not just as appealing to "greenies" but also as a thoughtful conservative's issue. The largest meeting of Heads of State in history, the Earth Summit, took place in Rio de Janeiro in 1992 and three international conventions—climate change, biodiversity (on which I was consulted) and desertification—came into existence.

But three things changed. First, there now are three times as many people alive today as when I was born and each new person deserves a minimum quality of life. Second, the sense of frugality was succeeded by a growing appetite for affluence and an overall attitude of entitlement. And third, conservative political advisors found advantage in demonizing the environment as comity vanished from the political dialogue.

Insufficient progress has brought humanity and the environment to a crisis state. The CO_2 level in the atmosphere at 415 ppm (parts per million) is way beyond a non-disruptive level around 350 ppm. (The pre-industrial level was 280 ppm.)

Human impacts on nature and biodiversity are not just confined to climate change. Those impacts will not produce just a long slide of continuous degradation. The pandemic is a direct result of intrusion upon, and destruction of, nature as well as wild-animal trade and markets. The scientific body of the UN Convention on Biological Diversity warned in 2020 that we could lose a million species unless there are major changes in human interactions with nature.

We still can turn those situations around. Ecosystem restoration at scale could pull carbon back out of the atmosphere for a soft landing at 1.5 degrees of warming (at 350 ppm), hand in hand with a rapid halt in production and use of fossil fuels. The Amazon tipping point where its hydrological cycle would fail to provide enough rain to maintain the forest in southern and eastern Amazonia can be solved with major reforestation. The oceans' biology is struggling with increasing acidity, warming and ubiquitous pollution with plastics: addressing climate change can lower the first two and efforts to remove plastics from our waste stream can improve the latter.

Indisputably, we need a major reset in our economies, what we produce, and what we consume. We exist on an amazing living planet, with a biological profusion that can provide humanity a cornucopia of benefits—and more that science has yet to reveal—and all of it is automatically recyclable because nature is very good at that. Scientists have determined that we can, in fact, feed all the people on the planet, and the couple billion more who may come, by a combination of selective improvements of productivity, eliminating food waste and altering our diets (which our doctors have been advising us to do anyway).

The Resetting Our Future series is intended to help people think about various ways of economic and social rebuilding that will support humanity for the long term. There is no single way to do this and there is plenty of room for creativity in the process, but nature with its capacity for recovery and for recycling can provide us with much inspiration, including ways beyond our current ability to imagine.

Ecosystems do recover from shocks, but the bigger the shock, the more complicated recovery can be. At the end of the Cretaceous period (66 million years ago) a gigantic meteor slammed into the Caribbean near the Yucatan and threw up so much dust and debris into the atmosphere that much of biodiversity perished. It was *sayonara* for the dinosaurs; their only surviving close relatives were precursors to modern day birds. It certainly was not a good time for life on Earth.

The clear lesson of the pandemic is that it makes no sense to generate a global crisis and then hope for a miracle. We are lucky to have the pandemic help us reset our relation to the Living Planet as a whole. We already have building blocks like the United Nations Sustainable Development Goals and various environmental conventions to help us think through more effective goals and targets. The imperative is to rebuild with humility and imagination, while always conscious of the health of the living planet on which we have the joy and privilege to exist.

Dr. Thomas E. Lovejoy is Professor of Environmental Science and Policy at George Mason University and a Senior Fellow at the United Nations Foundation. A world-renowned conservation biologist, Dr. Lovejoy introduced the term "biological diversity" to the scientific community.

Introduction

If you're reading this, chances are you've been suffering from the devastating fallout of the COVID-19 pandemic. Maybe it's lingering symptoms of a COVID infection, grief over the loss of loved ones, or struggling with loneliness and isolation. The pandemic has turned our world upside down in previously unimaginable ways. We're suffering as a human race in ways we have not felt for a very, very long time. But what if there is a way to use this pandemic to change things for the better? Certainly, we have fractious division as a result of COVID, but we have also seen people come together and help one another in wonderful ways that highlight the best aspects of humanity. What if the pandemic can help us – all of us – to reset the way we deal with suffering, as a person and as all of humanity?

Specifically, it is my aim to help you redefine your pain— whether it's emotional, physical, or both—so you can live a rich, vital, and meaningful life while you overcome seemingly insurmountable obstacles and build your future. The following pages contain practical tools that have the potential to transform your present experience, and ultimately your life. This may sound like an unrealistic claim, but I've seen the powerful and profound effect Acceptance and Commitment Therapy (ACT, said as one word) has had on my clients. I'm hopeful that this scientifically supported psychological approach will help you, too.

What should you expect to get out of reading this book? Well, I hope it's nothing short of a transformative experience that sets you on the path to a rich, vital, and meaningful life. These are big expectations, of course. My own experience with these kinds of books is that while I may not find *everything* in them to be of use, I almost always find *something* in them that is. Even if that's the most you get out of reading this, I will have, in some small way, done my job.

While I originally developed this material for people suffering from Lyme disease and chronic illness, I felt it was urgent to revise it for you. The physical and mental toll of the pandemic has been devastating—illness, loss, grief, overwork, overwhelm, isolation, disconnection, unemployment, fear, worry, relationship struggles—the list goes on. Whatever your difficulties may be, ACT was designed to help you deal with your immediate suffering, improve your functioning, increase your quality of life, and meet challenges with more resilience.

I want to be clear that while I might refer broadly to "your pandemic-related pain" in this book, I absolutely do not consider your specific circumstances to be generic, commonplace, or any less distressing than someone else's. The bottom line is that things aren't how you want them to be and you're suffering. The pandemic has profoundly affected your ability to live the life you want to live. This book will help you reclaim your life *right now* (as soon as Chapter 3).

Much of what's in this book is built on material generated by the top-notch behavioral scientists who founded ACT, particularly Steve Hayes and Russ Harris who have been generous in their permission to include versions of many of their techniques and exercises. I've put my own spin on things and my co-author has provided her firsthand experiences, but almost everything in the following pages has its roots in the work of others, specifically behavioral scientists and the ACT community of professionals who willingly share ideas and support the advancement of the science. (Please see the Recommended Reading.) I am standing on the shoulders of proverbial giants here, and I am eternally grateful to them. I urge you to seek out their ACT resources if you find the information in this book valuable.

While I didn't create ACT, I have been trained in it, I use it with my clients, and I try my best to practice and use it in my own life. Like most people, I'm not always successful, but that's okay. Be gentle with yourself. Change doesn't always come easily. Nevertheless, in my practice, I've seen the powerful and profound effects ACT has had on my clients. I'm hopeful that you too will have a life-changing experience using the ACT tools and that they will help you improve the quality of your life as you navigate the future.

Before we begin, there are several important points for you to keep in mind as we move forward on this journey together:

- It is critically important to understand that I am not a medical doctor and this is not a "Long Haul COVID Cure" book. The fact is, we are watching the science around this virus unfold in real time. As such, I urge you to seek reliable sources and stay informed as things evolve. While ACT is a scientifically supported treatment approach that has been helpful to people with similar issues, it has not been specifically tested on people with COVID. Hopefully, these data will be forthcoming. In the meantime, I hope this can be of help to you.

- There are two voices in this book. One a clinical psychologist (Joe) and the other a sufferer of the COVID infection (Julie) who will share her story, illustrating how her use of the ACT approach has benefitted her.

- I recommend reading this book in order, at least once, to get the full picture of the ACT model. After you have a grasp on the material, you can easily use this book as a reference guide, returning to parts that might be useful in the moment.

- While you may be tempted to simply read the exercises and not actually do them, I encourage you to engage as much as you can. You can probably get something out of just reading them, but with ACT, the more you do, the more you'll get out of it.

- Some books are meant to be read, others are meant to

be experienced, and this book is the latter. So take your time, read, re-read, savor, and experience it. I wrote this book from a place of compassion, and I hope that shows in obvious ways. But turning it over in your head and your heart a few times might help you connect with that intention.

- I also ask that you read this book with patience and an open mind. The ACT model is a bit paradoxical. It challenges preconceived notions and presents some ideas and approaches that may feel unfamiliar or unexpected to you at first. Please, read on and see where it goes. You might be pleasantly surprised at where you end up.

This can't be overstated: You deserve to live a rich, fulfilling, meaningful life *right now* in this moment—today, tomorrow, and for the rest of your life. It is my sincere belief that what follows in the pages of this book will help you do just that. I invite you to join me and reclaim your future from the COVID-19 pandemic.

Chapter 1

Welcome to ACT

When life kicks you, let it kick you forward.
—Kay Yow

We're All in This Together

As I write these words, the whole world is still in the grip of COVID-19—living with illness, fear, and uncertainty. For millions, there has been untold pain, loss, and suffering. The pandemic has caused major life changes on so many levels, compromising our physical, mental, social, familial, and economic health. The burdens are widespread and persistent from acute illness, long haul illness, unemployment, isolation, separation, quarantine, caretaking, poverty, overwork, grief, interpersonal friction, reduced opportunities, divorce, financial crises, economic instability, and the loss of social support. This list and the suffering go on and on.

Practically speaking, we have a tough road to navigate moving forward and rebuilding our lives. However, if we've learned anything from the pandemic, it's that when individuals approach adversity wisely, we are all elevated. This begs the question, how do we face our own individual challenges with resilience? As it turns out, ACT was developed specifically to answer this question. It can help you take control of the things over which you have some influence.

If the pandemic in general or the COVID-19 virus specifically has turned your life upside down, you may have found yourself putting everything on hold until it's over, until you're feeling better, until things are back to normal. It's natural to think this way. But what if there's not a "normal" to return to? With ACT you can navigate this uncharted territory, improve the quality of your life, and lead a richer, more vital, and more meaningful life despite the chaos, pain, illness, or uncertainty the pandemic has caused. If each of us can do this, the broadening effect of the ACT approach gains power and helps us transform how we experience pain and suffering.

People who are living in turmoil caused by the pandemic need ACT because it was designed exactly for situations over which we have little or no control.

It's Called ACT for a Reason

ACT was designed to help you move forward and live your life to the best of your ability right now, this very moment, despite the fallout of the pandemic—painful and devastating as it may be. At its core, ACT is about dealing with human suffering. More specifically, it's about creating a different relationship with whatever pain and difficulties you have. Rather than continuously struggling to avoid or vanquish your pain, ACT will help you co-exist with it while you take action to lead a fulfilling life no matter what your circumstances are.

As you may already intuitively know, the worst struggles we experience do not come from challenging situations or events. Instead, the greatest difficulties in our lives come from our attempts to avoid or escape discomfort, both physical and emotional. This is called experiential avoidance, and it's a natural part of our survival instinct. Unfortunately, it can lead to maladaptive and dysfunctional behavior, causing more problems than it prevents (Hayes et al, 2012). When we become so focused on avoiding pain, we end up not actually living our lives at all but expending our energy trying to be pain-free. This simply isn't realistic or possible.

A classic example is the alcoholic who drinks to avoid difficult emotions. Simply choosing to experience pain would be much less destructive than the havoc and damage wrought by excessive drinking and avoidance. Or maybe you know the kind of worker who expends so much energy pretending to be productive that it would be easier to do the actual job (and far less alienating and damaging in the long run). Of course, you don't have to be dependent on alcohol or avoid your job responsibilities to be excessively avoidant. We try to escape pain in countless ways. We watch too much TV, we stay in bad relationships, and we engage excessively with technology to avoid our feelings, put off purposeful action, and sidestep the discomforts of real human contact. We let our fluctuating emotions make our decisions, we keep others at a distance with our anger or irritability, and we become stingy with our talents for fear of embarrassment.

ACT asks us to let go of the idea that we can or should live pain-free lives. If we accept that we'll experience pain, we can

---

The Advent of ACT: ACT has been over 30 years in the making and is considered part of the "third wave" of behavioral therapies (Hayes et al, 2012). It's grounded in an extremely well-researched model called Relational Frame Theory, which focuses on how our minds form relations and use symbols and language to make connections in our mental processes. This is a remarkably adaptive human skill that can sometimes get us stuck in negative feedback loops. ACT is also part of a larger movement of psychotherapeutic approaches called Contextual Behaviorism (Hayes et al, 2013), specifically Functional Contextualism. Simply put, this is about doing what works (what is functional), when and where it works (in context). Functional Contextual approaches refuse to judge or categorize behavior outside the context in which the behavior occurs and without understanding the function of the behavior (Biglan and Hayes, 1996).

transform our suffering. This is a counterintuitive but powerful approach to life. It might not immediately feel comfortable, but it will eventually help you lead a more functional life if you're willing to try something different.

Pain is a part of the human experience. Suffering is a result of how we deal with pain. Our attempts to avoid pain lead to suffering.

Julie's Introduction to ACT Story

I learned about ACT in 2016 as an early editor of Dr. Joseph J. Trunzo's book *Living Beyond Lyme*, about coping with a devastating illness amidst medical confusion. I immediately started using the tools, which wasn't difficult. At the time I had a chronic condition that was certain to end in death. It's called Aging. (I'm joking, but only a little.)

Something that's terrible for your aging brain is rumination, and I ruminate. I'm aware of this, as is everyone who knows me well and has tried to help with advice like, "stop overthinking things," "look on the bright side," or "have an attitude of gratitude." Nope, none of that worked. But ACT did. It's straightforward and practical, but also elegantly designed. You'll see.

I don't have any special skills, and I didn't have any professional help applying ACT. I'm just a person who read a book and whose life is better for it, even after I got sick, lost my job, and ended up in the hospital with a COVID-19-related condition. At the end of each chapter I'll show you how I used ACT and how I fumbled it (and recovered).

While the anecdotes are mine, all of the advice in this book is from Dr. Trunzo (Joe, to me). He's a smart, deeply compassionate, dryly funny person and one of my oldest, dearest friends. He's also an extremely ethical, caring, and scientifically-minded professional who truly believes you're an extraordinary human being living under extraordinary circumstances in extraordinary times. If this doesn't shine through, it's because this book is an abbreviated version, my edit, of his original work. However, it was tailored specifically for you, from a place of genuine concern for your well-being, to help you navigate your own personal pandemic-related hardships as you build your future.

Chapter 2

ACT—How It Works

Do you want to know who you are? Don't ask. Act! Action will delineate and define you.
—Thomas Jefferson

Increase Psychological Flexibility

ACT is focused on giving you tools to reduce your suffering by increasing your psychological flexibility. This will allow you to stay in the moment, feel what you feel when you feel it, and take values-based actions. In short, ACT helps you to make meaningful decisions and fully experience the moments of your life under any circumstances.

Psychological Flexibility: The ability to *contact the present moment* more fully as a conscious human being and to *change or persist in behavior to serve valued ends* (Hayes et al, 2012).

Psychological Inflexibility: Engaging in *avoidant behavior* to escape the present moment because it's painful or undesirable.

When you're psychologically flexible, you're aware of and in touch with whatever experiences you're having, especially emotionally, at each moment in time (*contact with the present moment*). Your decisions are NOT based on attempts to avoid pain or discomfort but ARE based on what will move you toward what you truly value (*change or persist in behavior to serve valued ends*) regardless of your emotional or physical experiences. A psychologically flexible person is able to stay in contact with the present even if that present is uncomfortable, difficult, or painful.

To help develop psychological flexibility, ACT has identified six core processes designed to make you more Open, Centered, and Engaged. They are:

1. Defusion (Open)
2. Acceptance (Open)
3. Self-as-Context (Centered)
4. Contact with the Present Moment (Centered)
5. Values (Engaged)
6. Committed Action (Engaged)

The core processes work together to increase your psychological flexibility. The following overview will give you an idea of the purpose of each. For now, just take it in without worrying about how to be open, centered, and engaged. After you have a general sense of the processes, each chapter has specific exercises to help you firmly grasp and improve these skills.

Open Up with Defusion and Acceptance

Being open is about freeing yourself from the struggle to avoid, extinguish, enhance, or otherwise control your emotions. Instead, it asks you to fully experience your moment-to-moment thoughts and feelings without trying to control them. When you open up like this, you'll be able to see that your thoughts and feelings are all transient and not a basis for sound decision-making. In fact, making decisions based on transient states leads to suffering.

Defusion helps us to observe our thought processes, recognize that thoughts are just thoughts, and make decisions about how to engage with them. We have the amazing ability to think about what we're thinking about. As you read these words, there's a verbal script running through your head commenting on what you're reading, adding to your to-do list, worrying about the future, and thinking about the past while also analyzing, evaluating, judging, criticizing, etc. We also tend to believe everything we think. When we do that, we become "fused" with our thoughts, which can lead to dysfunction. Defusion frees us and prevents our thoughts from dominating and dictating the experience of our lives.

Acceptance opens us up to fully experiencing the private events of our lives, both physically and emotionally, including illness and worry. The whole idea of acceptance is to *live well when you're not feeling well*. It asks you to allow yourself to feel whatever you're feeling—anxiety, depression, pain, despair—without defense or struggle. It's the antithesis of avoidance. Acceptance allows us to release our futile attempts at controlling our emotions so we can put that energy into values-based activities. ACT is not designed to help you feel *differently*, it is designed to help you *feel* differently.

Center Yourself with Contact with the Present Moment and Self-as-Context

When you're centered, you're able to experience the moments of your life as they're happening, which is truly all we have. Circumstances often pull our thoughts into the past or the future, raising uncomfortable emotions like anxiety, regret, fear, and despair. But we can remove much of the fuel of these energy-draining emotions by remaining centered and focused on our experience of the moment.

Contact with the Present Moment, closely related to mindfulness, allows us to be psychologically present so we can fully and consciously connect and engage. While ACT recognizes that at times we must plan for the future and remember the past, it's beneficial for the majority of your life experience to be dominated by your connection to the present moment. In fact, it's the only aspect of our lives over which we can exert any control. As such, ACT promotes non-judgmental contact with the present experience of your life no matter how difficult, uncomfortable, painful, joyous, exhilarating, or devastating that feeling may be. In this space, you have more flexibility to make values-based decisions.

Self-as-Context is the point of view from which we can notice our thoughts, observe our lives, and make decisions about what to focus on. People who are suffering from misfortune have a tendency to over-identify with their experience. Because of this, your pandemic-related circumstances have the potential to overtake your life. By focusing on "who you were" and "hope to be again," you're rejecting your actual self in the process. In other words, you're defining yourself by the *content* of your life rather than the *context*. The content of your life is

---

Mindfulness is a vitally important skill to develop, applicable to all of the ACT processes. However, because it's a centuries-old practice with deep roots, you may be familiar with a different interpretation of mindfulness. It is perhaps most associated with Zen Buddhism and for good reason. Most people's basic understanding of mindfulness is drawn from their knowledge of Asian cultures and Buddhist teachings. It's this Eastern influence that's been incorporated into Western psychotherapy approaches led by Jon Kabat-Zinn, Eckhart Tolle, and many others (Williams and Kabat-Zinn, 2013). However, mindfulness is often mistaken for religious practice. While it may be utilized in certain religious rituals or practices, ACT takes a secular approach. For our purposes, *mindfulness is simply about giving your full attention to your experience of the present moment.*

merely the environment in which your life is happening. If you view yourself in context, you can discover who you are now (a person experiencing hardship) rather than defining yourself by the content ("I'm sick"/"I'm unemployed"/"I'm overwhelmed"/"I'm lonely").

Engage with Values and Committed Action

ACT is ultimately about *doing*. Real change comes from engaging to the best of your ability. Waiting to live your life until problems pass or things change will only lead to more suffering. ACT encourages you to *act* regardless of the circumstances. This action may have elements of pain or discomfort, but in service of moving you forward in a valued direction, it's acceptable and may even be necessary.

Values are freely chosen by you and will guide your decisions, acting as a compass for the purposeful direction you take in life. Defining your values will enable you to make choices that are informed by what's truly important to you. At any given time, we are either making decisions that move us toward or keep us away from what matters to us. If you've been avoiding or chasing an emotional experience, then discovering your values and using them to make decisions will be a true relief. A values-driven life won't be free of pain, but it will be a richer, more meaningful existence.

Committed Action occurs when you connect your actions to your values without letting the fear of pain or discomfort affect your decisions. ACT asks that you take committed action toward your values at all times with full acknowledgement and acceptance of the fact that you may be exposed to difficult or uncomfortable emotions, feelings, or sensations. It's important to note that committed action is absolutely not habitual busyness. In many circumstances, relaxing or choosing NOT to do a particular thing is a perfectly valid "action." As your life becomes aligned with your values, you'll see how decisions are easier to make, action is easier to take, and fear is easier to accept.

Values-driven decisions and actions are an absolute necessity for progress, whatever your situation.

Visualize ACT

Taken as a whole, each of the core processes supports the others to improve psychological flexibility, allowing you to contact the present moment fully and make choices in the service of your chosen values. All of the ACT tools are connected and affected by the others. This visual representation of the model may seem daunting, but simply take it in for now and we'll revisit later.

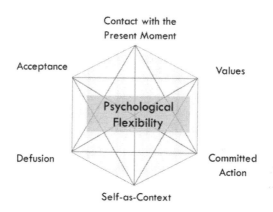

The Hexaflex Model of Psychological Flexibility
(reprinted with permission from Hayes et al, 2012)

Apply ACT to Your Pandemic Circumstances

ACT encourages you to engage in your life right now, no matter how difficult or painful it might be in the moment. Improving your psychological flexibility allows you to sidestep the "what ifs" of your future. Instead, ACT brings focus to your unique internal experience. While answering what-if questions may ultimately be important, you don't have to ignore your values, sacrifice all of your time, or put your life on hold until you get those answers. On the contrary, ACT encourages you to engage with your life to the fullest of your ability at *every* moment.

Julie's Pandemic Story

Like most people, I care about my family, friends, pets, hobbies, travel, work, and health. Your list might vary and you may pour a lot of energy into one thing, building your life around it. That's what I've done with travel. I have this in common with my husband, who also happens to be the most well-traveled person I know. He's traveled for work since I've known him, and three years ago I got a job doing the same. This took me all over the US, to places I never dreamed about, obscure pockets of the country, amazing spots I'd never think to pick for a vacation, and secure locations most civilians never see.

However, the downsides of a 100% travel job are many, and one is "travel crud." If an illness was out there, it'd be sitting next to me on the plane. So, I was worried about the reports of COVID-19 in the US. But it was so early in the pandemic when I got an unusual flu-like sickness, I only joked about it being the "Rona."

Then I developed severe chest pains that sent me to the hospital with an inflamed heart muscle caused by COVID-19 (most likely. That's as definitive a diagnosis as many of us will ever get). While I was recovering much too slowly, on lots of medications and fuzzy-brained, I was permanently laid off from my job. Over the course of weeks, everything had changed for the worse. I was in pain, fatigued, foggy, grounded, unemployed, dependent on others, and insecure about my future.

Chapter 3

Defusion—Don't Believe Everything You Think

There is nothing either good or bad, but thinking makes it so.
—**William Shakespeare**

Open Up with Defusion

Human beings are thinking creatures. We're always doing it—as we're talking, listening, writing, reading, running errands. Chances are, if we're conscious (and sometimes even not) that little voice constantly running in the back of our minds is active and vocal. There's nothing wrong with this. It's part of being human. However, we have a strong tendency to become fused with that voice and accept whatever our minds are telling us without question or doubt. It is, after all, *your* voice representing *your* thoughts, so how wrong could it be? As it turns out, it can often be quite problematic.

Defusion teaches us how to live comfortably with our internal dialogue and not give it dominion over our lives.

Understand Defusion

Looking at the content of your mind (your thinking self) is nothing new in psychology. It's a hallmark approach in Cognitive Behavioral Therapy (CBT) to call that voice out for being irrational and wrestle it back to a more rational place. Under a wide range of circumstances, this can be quite helpful. *But there is nothing irrational about your pandemic experience.* It's not the product of your thinking mind. It's the product of very real events caused by a virus. However, not allowing your thoughts to define your reality is a very important part of the process of being psychologically flexible.

Instead of examining our thoughts and asking if they're right or wrong, rational or irrational, healthy or unhealthy, ACT focuses on the *function* of our thoughts. To understand this, let's look at exactly what's happening when we think:

- Whenever you're thinking, you're using language.
- When you use language, you're using symbols (words).
- You use these symbols to create relations among the various events, objects, and emotions of your life.

Naturally, you connect the pandemic to the devastation it's brought to your life. In your mind, the pandemic, your life, and devastation become "related frames." These connections, accurate or not, have a tendency to stick.

Survival and Relational Frames: The connections our brains make have a long history of saving human lives. Imagine you're living in a world where you have to forage for food. You eat a berry off of a bush, and you get really sick. The berry-sickness relational frame will keep you from eating a berry from that bush again. But should it keep you from eating all berries from every bush forever?

Sometimes our relational frames get tangled up, especially when dealing with emotions. That entanglement, or fusion, prevents us from being able to observe our own thought process. In essence, it automates our response. As such, we end up behaving in accordance with those relational frames—we never eat any berries from any bushes at all. This inhibits us from being able to do things that might be good or necessary for our health and well-being—such as eating nutritious berries. If you remain fused with the fear-based thought that "berries will make me sick," you end up depriving yourself of the benefits of healthy berries.

Fusion with our thinking selves leads to significant dysfunction and experiential avoidance in our lives. Defusion will give you some separation from the stories you tell yourself so you can decide how to react. To do this, you first have to observe your thoughts. This is not about *controlling* or *stopping* your mind. That's a futile game, and it's not how our minds work. You can't push your thoughts out of your head, control them, or make them go away. And you don't have to. To borrow a phrase, *you can't control your thoughts; you can only control your reactions to them*. And when you don't engage with unhelpful thoughts, over time they will become less disruptive.

Try Defusion Now: Defusion can be used effectively right now, in this moment, no matter how distressed or sick you might feel. To defuse from your thoughts, you will be consciously creating some separation between your thinking self and your observing self. We generally live as the thinker. But it's the observer who can step back and listen to your thoughts and the stories you tell yourself. To get into the mindset of the observer, you will simply acknowledge that you're having a thought and allow it to exist without judgment or struggle. In other words, have whatever thoughts you're having, but observe the fact that you're having them and carry them with you lightly while you forge ahead and do what really matters to you (Wilson and DuFrene, 2010). Here's how:

1. Take a moment to reflect on what your mind is telling you about your life since the pandemic hit. Make a list, and feel free to get as specific as you can about what you're truly thinking. Here are some general examples you can expand on if they resonate with you: I can't do the things I love anymore. I'm overwhelmed all the time. I'm a burden to the people I care about.

2. To get into the mind of the observer, choose one of your thoughts from the list. I'll use *I can't do the things I love*

anymore. Take a moment to experience your feelings about this thought, intensely unpleasant as they may be.

3. Now, label the thought as a thought: *I'm having the thought* that I can't do the things I love anymore.

4. Go deeper into the perspective of the observer with: *I notice* that I'm having the thought that I can't do the things I love anymore.

5. Treat your mind, your thinking self, as a separate entity with: *My mind is telling me* that I can't do the things I love anymore.

6. Again, take a moment and experience how these new statements make you feel. If you notice that the shift in language has distanced you from your emotional experience, you've successfully defused!

Remember that your thoughts are connected symbolic representations based on the experiences of your life. Words might be sophisticated symbols, but they're symbols nonetheless. Thinking of them as such will give you a little distance and allow you to identify the connections (relational frames) you've made between your thoughts and experiences. For example, the symbols in *I can't do the things I love anymore* connect the pandemic and the activities you enjoy. If you simply recognize that the connection is only symbolic and need not dominate your experience of the present moment, then you give yourself the opportunity to defuse from the thought and respond with flexibility.

Find Your Distressing Thoughts: Some of the stories we tell ourselves are so ingrained that it's hard to see them for what they are. If you're having trouble, try the following to identify your distressing thoughts:

• **Write It Down**: Distressing thoughts can be sneaky. One way to catch them is to stay alert during your day and write your distressing thoughts down when they arise (Hayes et al, 1999). Simply carrying them around with you while you go on with your day can act as a powerful metaphor, showing you how distressing thoughts can co-exist with values-driven action. This will help you see that you're more than your immediate, temporary, transient thoughts.

- **Greatest Hits**: Does that thought sound familiar? There's a good chance a thought is one of your Greatest Hits if you can classify it as "the same old story" (Hayes et al, 1999). Most people have them, and many of them have deep roots—*I'm not good enough, people don't like me, I'm too worried to be any good to anyone, bad things always happen to me.* When you find them, take some time to defuse from these old thoughts you've been playing on repeat.

- **Rules**: Rule-governed thinking includes any statements that contain *should, must, ought,* or *if-then* language. *I should be doing more right now. If I were less stressed, then I'd be a better parent. I ought to be feeling better.* Rule-governed thought patterns are inflexible and lend themselves to suffering (Harris, 2009).

- **Reasons**: If you find yourself coming up with excuses for not engaging in values-driven behavior, this is reason-governed thinking. *I can't take better care of myself because I'm too stressed. I can't be there for my family because I don't feel well. I can't do the things I care about because I'm so busy.* This kind of reason-governed thinking could hold you back from making meaningful life choices (Harris, 2009).

- **Judgments**: Negative or positive judgments of others or yourself often lead to fused thinking, self-fulfilling prophecies, disappointments, and inflexibility in your thought processes and behaviors (Harris, 2009). *I'll always be in pain. The pandemic will ruin my life forever. Other people are successful and happy right now.* These are all examples of unhelpful judgments.

- **Past and Future**: Fusion with positive or negative thoughts regarding the past or future compromises your ability to be flexible. If you're stuck in your thoughts about your past "good" life and convinced your future will be consumed by the negative fallout of the pandemic, this can paralyze your present (Harris, 2009).

- **Self-Stories**: Thoughts you have about yourself are essentially stories you made up based on interpretations of your past experiences. *I'm sick. I'm overwhelmed. I'm tired. I'm tough.* Whatever the story may be, it lends itself to inflexibility in the present moment when your situation may call for an approach that's different from your conceptualized self (Harris, 2009).

When you are opened up to your thoughts, you can decide if they have functional merit. With the ability to observe our thoughts comes the ability to decide how much or how little we want to engage with those thoughts. Defusion is not concerned with whether a thought is right or wrong, correct or incorrect, rational or irrational. Again, in ACT, what matters is *function*. So, ask yourself if the thought will help you move toward what you value or away from it. If it's useful, engage away! If not, defuse from it.

Thanks, Mind! A popular technique for defusing from distressing thoughts is to consciously dismiss them when they come up. (*I don't have to listen to my mind right now.*) You can thank your mind for making you aware. (*Thanks, mind!*) And you can tell it that you don't want to attend to that right now (*That's not important.*) (Hayes et al, 1999).

Practice Defusion

We've believed our thoughts for our whole lives, so defusion is tricky. Because of this, ACT practitioners have come up with a lot of ways to help. The following metaphors and exercises are only a small sample of what's available, but they should give you an excellent foundation for creating separation between your thinking self and your observing self.

Pick from a Menu: Treat your thoughts like a drop down menu on your computer. You don't have any control over what items show up, but you do get to choose which option to click. This choice is based on the action you want your computer to perform. You don't spend time trying to get rid of the other menu options—you let them exist while you choose the one that will get you where you want to go.

You can do the same thing with your thoughts. At any given point in time, you probably have several different thoughts running through your mind. *I'm unlovable* is right next to *I love my family. I can't exercise like I used to* is near *I value my health. I'm lonely* is on the flipside of *I treasure my friendships*. Use the "drop down menu" to pick the thoughts to engage with based on your valued outcome. Let the others simply exist with minimal impact on your life, because they don't have to have an impact if you don't engage with them.

Similarly, when you go to a restaurant, you don't write the menu, just like you don't control your thoughts. You look over the menu and pick what you want, letting the other menu items exist as they are. You don't contact the chef and demand to have an item removed because you don't like it. You don't negotiate with the waitstaff to rename a sandwich. You simply let the menu exist and engage with the items that you want based on what you value—health, taste, novelty, familiarity, budget. Treat your thoughts similarly. You don't have to buy into every thought you have in the same way that you don't have to buy every item on a menu at a restaurant.

Getting Hooked: A phrase that's often used to describe fusion with your thoughts is "getting hooked" (Whitney, 2013, in Stoddard and Afari, 2014), which leads us to this fly fishing metaphor. Skilled fly fishers tie realistic fake flies and manipulate their movements on the water's surface so well that the fish can't distinguish actual flies from bait. The trout buys that the fake fly is real, bites, and gets hooked.

Your mind is a skilled fly fisher, making up thoughts and tempting you with them until you take the bait and get hooked. The more you struggle, the deeper the hook goes. However, your mind can only tie flies on barbless hooks. It feels like you can't escape, but if you pause from the struggle and spit out the hook, you're free. Your mind is constantly presenting you with excellent bait, but you don't have to take it. Even if you do, you can stop and spit out the hook at any time.

The Silly Ones: There are several techniques to enhance defusion that many would consider to be lacking in seriousness. But a big part of defusion is about not taking your thoughts too seriously. So, tapping into some silliness can be helpful.

- **Repetition**: Repeat your thoughts to yourself over and over again until they sound like nonsense.
- **Sing-Song**: Sing your distressing thoughts to various tunes—childhood songs work well (Hayes et al, 1999). Or use an app to turn your voice recording into a song.
- **Bullies**: Treat your thoughts like bullies and remind yourself that you're in charge, not your mind. Say to your mind what you would say to that bully—feel free to use colorful language if it helps!
- **Voices**: Use silly voices, like those of your favorite cartoon characters, to say your distressing thoughts.
- **Slow-Mo**: Say your distressing or uncomfortable thoughts very, very slowly—make it painfully slow—to the point where you become bored with the thought itself and it

loses its weight. *I... am... not... good... enou... oh, forget it.*

Although some of these ideas may seem simple, you'll only know what works for you if you try them. If you're thinking that these "silly ones" aren't for you, challenge yourself to defuse from that thought and try them anyway. These techniques don't take a lot of effort, and you might find yourself laughing about previously dire or devastating thoughts. When that happens, you've successfully defused!

Experiential Ones: Experiential based defusion exercises are also helpful (Hayes et al, 2012). They're all about leaning in to your experiences, really feeling what you're feeling, and going through the storm to get out.

- **Sink into Discomfort**: This technique is critical in dealing with anxiety. When people immerse themselves in activities that terrify them, they eventually become less scared. To do this, really concentrate on your distressing thoughts. Then remind yourself that they're only thoughts and it's possible to act contrary to them. In fact, you probably pull this off every day of your life. Have you ever thought, *I can't stand that person*, but were polite and civil anyway? If so, you acted in a way that was inconsistent with your thinking. That's defusion. Whenever you do something that's not dictated by your thoughts (*I dislike her*) but by your values (*I treat others well*), this is movement in the right direction.

- **Concede the Argument**: Acknowledge that your thought is correct. *My mind is telling me that things will never be the same. Fine mind, you're right, so what am I going to do about it?* Giving up the struggle, much like letting go of the rope in a tug of war, frees you up to focus on doing what matters rather than continuing to struggle with your mind. You can choose to be right or choose to live fully. Given the choice in any situation, what's your preference? If you refuse to argue and use "you're right" as a cue to action, you increase the likelihood that you'll move forward.

- **Walk with Your Mind**: You can do this with a trusted friend, therapist, or alone using a tape recorder. Walk around the room and have your friend, therapist, or your recorded voice repeat your distressing and troubling thoughts over and over while you're doing other things. This reinforces the reality that you can be functional and do things while uncomfortable thoughts are rattling around in your head.

- **Be Mindful**: Mindfulness shows itself in all of the core processes of ACT, so being mindful can absolutely help with defusion (Hayes et al, 2012). Remember that being mindful simply means *giving your full attention to your experience of the present moment*. If you commit to a mindful, open approach to life, you're less likely to fuse with thoughts and have them guide your behavior. Similarly, if you engage in open mindfulness—watching your thoughts as external objects without any specific use—you can facilitate the separation you're seeking between your thinking and observing selves.

Visualizations: The following visualization exercises will help you stay grounded in the present while giving you useful metaphors you can call on as needed.

- **Dandelions in the Wind:** This mindfulness exercise is a variation of a rather famous metaphor called "Leaves on a Stream" (Hayes et al, 1999). It was further utilized by ACT icon Russ Harris (2009). "Leaves on a Stream" is widely available in many published works and in various places online. This is a version I frequently use that I think creates a nice platform for dealing with difficult thoughts:

Sit in a comfortable position and either close your eyes or rest them gently on a fixed spot in the room. Take several easy breaths, paying close attention to the sensation of the air moving in and out of your lungs. After a few moments, visualize yourself sitting in a peaceful field. The dandelions are going to seed, and a gentle wind is blowing. As the breeze flows, it carries the wispy dandelion tufts along with it.

For the next few minutes, imagine each thought that enters your mind as one of those dandelion seeds. Let the breeze carry them along lightly in the air. Do this with each thought—pleasurable, painful, or neutral. Even if you have joyous or enthusiastic thoughts, imagine they're dandelion wisps and let them float by. If your thoughts momentarily stop, continue to watch the wisps float on by in the breeze. Sooner or later, your thoughts will start up again. Allow the breeze to blow at its own pace. Don't try to speed it up and rush your thoughts along. You're not trying to hurry the dandelion seeds or "get rid" of your thoughts. You're simply allowing them to come and go at their own pace.

If your mind says, this is dumb, I'm bored, or I'm not doing this right, place those thoughts on the dandelion wisps too. Let them float away in the breeze. If a wisp hovers or gets stuck, allow it to hang around until it gets caught up in the breeze. If the thought comes up again, watch it pass by again. If a difficult or painful feeling arises, acknowledge it. Say to yourself, I notice myself having a feeling of boredom/ impatience/frustration. See those thoughts as dandelions and allow them to float along. From time to time, your thoughts may hook you and distract you from being fully present in this exercise. This is normal. As soon as you realize you've become sidetracked, gently bring your attention back to the visualization exercise.

With practice, you'll get to the point where you can pretty

easily visualize putting difficult or uncomfortable thoughts on dandelion tufts and letting them blow away with the breeze without judgment or struggle.

- **Boat on the Water**: A similar exercise to "Leaves on the Stream" or "Dandelions in the Wind" is "Boat on the Water" (Bryan, 2013; in Stoddard and Afari, 2014). Rather than placing thoughts on objects and watching them float away, you experience the rise and fall of thoughts as if you were on a boat.

   Imagine you're in a boat on the ocean. Engage all of your senses as you float along. Smell the ocean air. Feel the sun on your skin. Picture the horizon. Feel the boat swaying beneath you. Gentle waves begin to hit the boat. You feel it rise and fall as you hear each small wave lap against the hull. Almost as soon as you realize a wave has come, it passes. It's not long before another comes along. Sometimes the waves come quickly and powerfully then pass. Sometimes the waves seem so big they're all you can see, until they too pass. As the waves continuously go past you—some big, some small—feel each one. And as you do, try to notice any thoughts or feelings that arise. As you notice these internal experiences, see if you can simply ride the waves, allowing the thoughts and feelings to rise and fall, come and go. If you get swept overboard, simply recognize this, climb back in the boat, and continue to ride the waves.

This exercise helps you tap into the transient nature—the rise and fall—of difficult thoughts and emotions. You can't control your thoughts any more easily than you can control the waves of the ocean. But you can allow the waves to happen, to come and go, as they will.

When you use any of the above techniques—silly voices, songs, characters, dandelion tufts—you're creating different relational frames for your difficult thoughts. The more you do this, the greater the distance you put between your thinking self and your observing self. This separation gives you more room for psychological flexibility, which is the goal.

Apply Defusion to Your Painful Pandemic Thoughts

Defusion is about recognizing your thoughts for what they are—connected symbolic representations based on the experiences of your life. There's no need to judge them or struggle against them. In fact, the more you do that, the worse things will tend to go for you.

You'll certainly have thoughts about your pandemic-related circumstances that need to be attended to—thoughts that will help you solve practical problems and move you in valued directions in your life. But there will also be times when your mind feeds you information that isn't particularly helpful. It's not out to get you, but it's not perfect either.

Remember, thoughts aren't good or evil, right or wrong, healthy or unhealthy—they just are. Instead of judging their merits, evaluate them by their function. Ask yourself if engaging with a particular thought—at the moment, in context—will help you move your life forward in a valued direction. If not, defuse—float it away, pick another menu item, thank your mind—and move on.

Julie's Defusion Story

After my hospital stay, even simple tasks were exhausting. (I had to take a break in the middle of making myself a cup of tea!) So, I was nervous when I finally decided I could manage an easy walk. I picked a flat gravel loop through the woods, the path I took to give my dog some exercise when I was phoning it in. It was slow going, and I was worried I'd run out of steam halfway around. On top of dreading the idea that I might have to sit on a stump in the woods while my concerned husband watched me catch my breath, I was also beating myself up:

This is terrible (judgment). *If I'd worked out more when I was well, I'd be further along now* (rules/past fixation). *I'm never going to be able to hike, travel, run around like I used to* (reasons/future fixation).

I'd like to say I immediately recognized that none of these thoughts were useful, but I didn't. After I vented to my husband, I was still mad even though I knew I was ruining a perfectly nice walk. So, I tried defusion. I like to start by agreeing with myself, because I love it when I'm right—*this* **is** *terrible!* Then I use the basic defusion language trick—*I'm having the thought that this is terrible. I'm having the thought...* and done!

This almost always instantly works for me. Here's why. When I say to myself, *this is terrible*, my mind agrees (because I'm right). And when I say to myself, *I'm having the thought that this is terrible*, my mind agrees (right again!), only now it's agreeing with the fact that I'm having a thought. When I think, *I notice I'm having the thought*, my mind agrees that I'm noticing (yes, I am).

If one of these thoughts pops up again, I go silly. For me, the most effective one is to speak slowly. *I... should... have...* That's as far as I get before I give up because I can be impatient (which is partly why the slow walk was annoying in the first place).

Julie's Tip: Joe and other ACT practitioners highly encourage users to come up with their own brain hacks for all of the processes. I'm perfectly happy with the existing ones, but eventually some of my own tricks emerged. While *I'm having the thought* is nothing short of genius and I'll never stop using it, I'll also agree with myself using the improvisation principle, *Yes, and*. It validates my bad premise and leads me to a better idea. Plus, I think it's funny to imagine my dysfunctional thoughts as comedy setups.

Chapter 4

Acceptance—We Are Always Whole

Acceptance doesn't mean resignation; it means understanding that something is what it is and that there's got to be a way through it.
—**Michael J. Fox**

Open Up with Acceptance

Of all of the concepts in ACT, acceptance is the one people struggle with the most, simply because it's the most widely misunderstood. It is also arguably the most important and may hold the key to living a better life than you're living right now. Since there are a lot of common misunderstandings about acceptance, it's important to first be clear about what it does not mean:

- *Acceptance is NOT* giving up or moving on.
- *Acceptance is NOT* "pulling yourself up by your boot-straps."
- *Acceptance is NOT* tolerating your difficult situation.
- *Acceptance is NOT* "sucking it up."
- *Acceptance is absolutely NOT* approval of what's happening.

No one is asking you to feel great about your circumstances or think that it's the best thing that's ever happened to you. People often assume that the process of accepting something means you're inherently approving of it or that it has to become a "good thing" in your life. That could not be further from the truth.

Acceptance has an ancient history rooted in Eastern philosophy and religion. Many modern psychotherapy approaches have embraced varying definitions of acceptance as core parts of their therapeutic models. However, for our purposes, ACT defines acceptance as "the voluntary adoption of an intentionally open, receptive, flexible, and non-judgmental posture with respect to moment-to-moment experience" (Hayes et al, 2012). To clarify:

- *Acceptance IS* being open to the full range of experiences that your life has to offer, both pleasant and unpleasant.
- *Acceptance IS* embracing the reality that there will be difficulty and pain as well as happiness, joy, and everything in between.
- *Acceptance IS* having the willingness and flexibility to live your life as fully as possible despite your circumstances.

In our culture, we're constantly sold the idea that we're supposed to be happy or feeling great all the time, and if we're not then something's wrong with us. Since we don't want something to be wrong with us, we try to avoid things we think will make us unhappy in the futile attempt to prevent unpleasant emotions, sensations, or difficulties. The word futile is used purposefully here. While experiential avoidance may be an effective strategy to hide from unpleasant emotions in the short term, in the long term it's impossible to live a life free of unpleasant emotional experiences. It simply isn't human.

The real cause of suffering in people's lives is not the pain they experience—from illness, anxiety, depression, loneliness, insecurity, disappointment, or frustration—but their attempts to avoid that pain.

If experiential avoidance is the poison, then acceptance is the antidote. An absolute reality of life is that it inherently involves difficulty and pain. Of course, I would never ask anyone to put themselves in a painful situation if it's not moving them in a desired direction in their life, and you shouldn't ask this of yourself either. However, experiencing pain *in service of what you value* is a fundamental necessity and truism of human existence. In other words, if you're receptive to experiencing your full range of emotions, you have a much better chance of moving your life in a direction that's meaningful to you. Instead of struggling to avoid pain, you get to do what's really important to you, regardless of how you might feel.

Pain is a fundamental state of being human. Suffering is a choice that depends entirely on how we approach the pain in our lives.

Understand Acceptance

Acceptance asks us to remain open to experiencing all that life has to offer (or sometimes throws at us) no matter how difficult it might be. Much like it's futile to try not to think about something, it's equally futile to try not to feel something. The more we try not to feel, the more our lives get stuck. Moreover, when you spend your life in service of experiential avoidance (trying not to feel), it usually leads to suffering. However, if you're willing to open yourself up to the full range of human experiences, your life will no longer be hindered by this damaging control strategy.

Take a Ride on a Balloon: The experience of acceptance is a lot like flying in a hot air balloon. They both offer the potential of something beautiful—seeing the world in a totally different and fantastic way that's not easily available to you on a day-to-day basis. However, ballooning is also fraught with danger. While doing it with an experienced professional is a pretty safe activity, the fact of the matter is that you're high up in the air, subject to weather events, mechanical failure, and other flying objects. Anything could go wrong. But if you want the beautiful vistas, you have to *willingly choose* to accept the risk. If you choose not to accept the risk, you don't get to experience all of the beauty and joy the balloon ride has to offer. This mirrors the reality of life—if you don't accept that awful things can and sometimes will happen, your life will be less full, less meaningful, and less vital. It may be "safer," but at what cost?

Additionally, if you want to go anywhere in a balloon, you need to burn the fuel (feel the emotions). This is what fills the balloon and gives it lift. If you turn off the fuel (try to stop feeling the emotions) you'll be grounded, unable to go anywhere. But if you open up the flame and let the fuel burn—if you allow yourself to experience your emotions—the balloon (and your life) gets bigger and lighter. The next thing you know, you're on your way, which is what you wanted in the first place. Interestingly enough, no matter how much fuel you burn or how hot the air gets, hot air balloons don't burst. In fact, burning the fuel (again, feeling the emotions) allows you to fly higher. The hot air never becomes bigger than the balloon itself. Similarly, even though most of us are terrified of being overwhelmed by our emotions, they can never become bigger than you are.

You may have little control over where the wind takes you, but it's balloonist tradition to fly wherever, land wherever, and simply enjoy the journey for its own sake. Our own lives don't have to be quite so directionless and subject to the changing winds, but we all have times when attempts to control the direction or events of our lives takes a whole lot of effort but has little effect. ACT in general and acceptance specifically are much more about letting go and embracing the journey wherever it may it take us, as long as that journey is truly important to us.

It's probably easy to imagine accepting fear to take a balloon ride or to do something you chose to do. But you didn't choose to live through a pandemic, so how does any of this apply to what you're going through? As it happens, acceptance is at its greatest importance when things are thrust upon you over which you have no control.

Consider Viktor Frankl: During World War II, the psychiatrist Viktor Frankl was sent to several concentration camps where he was surrounded by unspeakable horrors and where his entire family, save his sister, died. Being the physician that he was, he did all he could to tend to the health and well-being of those suffering and dying around him. And he found meaning in this activity. When he was given the opportunity to move to a rest camp—to effectively alleviate much of his own suffering—he chose to stay in the concentration camp and continue to make his rounds and help those to whom he was tending. In this situation of tremendous pain and horror that was thrust upon him over which he had no control, he found a way to live meaningfully amidst his pain. So meaningfully, in fact, that when he had the opportunity to ease his own pain, to leave that horrible place, he chose to continue doing what was truly important to him. He chose to say "yes" to living in a concentration camp (Wilson and DuFrene, 2010).

Frankl had no choice about the origin of his pain. He could not easily solve his problems. But, by tapping into what he valued, by changing his relationship to his pain and suffering, he transformed himself and helped countless others in the process. Frankl was an extraordinary human being living under extraordinary circumstances in extraordinary times, *and so are you*!

We're built to experience a broad range of emotions, from extreme pain to pure joy. We can handle all of it. While it is human nature to try to avoid painful experiences, that will get us stuck. So, in order to do what you love, what's really important to you, you have to choose to accept that there are unpleasant aspects to your pursuit. If you decide to avoid unpleasantness, then you miss out on all of the pleasure and joy as well. They're two sides of the same coin. You can either keep the whole coin or throw it all away but throwing away the coin wouldn't make you immune to suffering.

If you open yourself up to experiencing all of your emotions and accept that there will be pain, you're free to engage in any activity you find meaningful. This is the reward of acceptance.

Practice Acceptance

There are many exercises out there for enhancing acceptance. Metaphors, like the balloon, will help you grasp the concepts. But ultimately, *you must engage in acceptance to build this skill.* And the more you practice, the better you'll get at it.

Passengers on the Bus: This classic ACT metaphor was designed to help you tap into the acceptance process (Hayes et al, 1999).

Imagine you're a bus driver. You're expected to keep your route and arrive at your stops on time. At each stop, passengers get on and off the bus. Some passengers are friendly, others are neutral, and some are downright mean. They yell things at you. They're smelly. And they make you feel uncomfortable. As the bus driver, what can you do? The unwelcome passengers paid their fare. They're not threatening to cause you or anyone else any harm, so it's not a safety issue. If you stop the bus and argue with them or try to throw them off, they'll probably refuse to leave. They have a right to public transportation. The more you fight and argue, the later you'll be in keeping to your route. If, however, you keep driving — letting the nasty passengers take the ride — you get to keep your schedule. And at some point, the troublesome passenger will get off the bus.

Thoughts, like bus passengers, come and go. The happy ones

and the distressing ones all get on and off the bus. If you allow that process to happen while you keep motoring along, you end up better off than if you stopped everything and fought or struggled with your distressing thoughts.

Give It Form: The following exercise is adapted largely from Russ Harris's work (2009). I recommend reading it through a few times to get the hang of the script. You could also record yourself, or someone else, to guide you through the exercise. Either way, don't worry too much about rigidly adhering to the script. This is a guide designed to help you create some separation between you and your experience. As long as you remain true to the overall spirit of the exercise, it doesn't matter if you miss a word or a sentence here or there. As with all mindfulness exercises, if you find yourself drifting, just gently acknowledge that and guide yourself back to the exercise.

Settle into a comfortable position. Close your eyes or focus on a specific point in the room. Take a few easy breaths. Notice how the breath feels as it goes in and out of your body... the coolness as it goes in and the warmth as it goes out. Stay in this space for a few minutes, focusing on your senses, what you hear, see, smell, and feel. If you find yourself drifting, gently acknowledge that and come back to your sensory experiences.

In a gentle and compassionate way, focus on what's distressing you. This may feel uncomfortable, but that's okay. Notice and sit with that feeling rather than pushing it away. With each breath, feel yourself expanding around that feeling and loosening up around it. Whatever the feeling is—sadness, anger, frustration, fear, pain—remain open to feeling it rather than running away from it or pushing it away. Breathe into it and expand around it. As you feel that discomfort, really try to attend to the feeling itself. In what part of your body does the feeling reside? Where do you experience it, where does it feel most intense? Focus on how it feels in that part of your body. Try to imagine what kind of shape or form it might have. Does it have a color? If you were to touch it, what would it feel like? Would it be warm or cold? Rough or smooth? Soft or hard? Notice all of these aspects of the feeling— observe them with curiosity. Touch the form of your feeling, imagine holding it in your hands, not altering or changing it, but simply holding it lightly and watching it. What does it do? It may get smaller or bigger. It may pulse or move. It may feel warm or cold. Notice and observe these things curiously. Recognize that even if the feeling gets bigger, no matter how big it gets, it doesn't get any heavier as you hold it. It doesn't consume or overtake you. It simply exists, doing its thing.

Now imagine dropping it or letting it go—not throwing or pushing it away. It may stay close to you. It may drift away a little bit and then come back. Notice what it does, how it exists. Attend to the feeling as it exists outside of you for a little bit. Do you notice how the feeling can be there and you can do other things? Your mind has probably drifted several times by now, so you know you can do other things while the feeling is there. Focus on that coexistence for a bit. After some time, allow the form to come back to you, to be part of you again. But notice if your experience of it has changed at all. Not whether the feeling has changed, but how your relationship with it may be different. Sit with that experience for a bit.

When you are ready, begin to focus on your senses again. Take a few more easy breaths, and soak in the experience.

After "giving it form," do you notice anything different about the feeling? When you give it some kind of form that you can visualize, it makes it easier to imagine it being outside of yourself and not dominating your life quite as much. You'll note that nothing in the exercise asked you to change your feeling. All you did was create a different perspective or relationship with it. At the end of the exercise, you were asked to allow the feeling back into your body because true acceptance means you choose to coexist with your present reality and all the associated feelings rather than struggling against them. This is an essential step to living a vital, meaningful life.

Apply Acceptance to Your Pandemic-Related Distress

Human beings are problem-solving machines. It's a wonderful gift we have that has made our world a far better and more comfortable place to be. However, problem solving is really only effective when we're dealing with *solvable problems*. Many issues you're struggling with now may not be solvable, at least not in an immediate sense, and your attempts to do so may have left you feeling deeply sad, angry, frustrated, or hopeless. If your intent is to "solve" your problem so you don't have to feel those emotions anymore, to make the unpleasantness go away, you're engaging in experiential avoidance, and this will likely not improve your life. In fact, it will probably get you stuck.

Acceptance can help. All it asks is that you be open to your unique, internal, private experiences. If you stop pouring energy into making pain and emotions go away, you just might create enough wiggle room to move toward something more rewarding and more valuable in your life. If you take the energy that you use trying not to *feel* (angry or sad or whatever) and put it into your kids, your partner, your friends, your work, a hobby—anything that really matters—this could help you have a better experience in the moment. Will acceptance make the sadness or anger go away? Most likely not. But it will stop your emotions from dictating your actions.

If you allow yourself to experience all of your feelings—if you don't invest yourself in fighting them off—you'll free yourself to engage in more meaningful activities. Of course, you may not be able to engage in a valued activity as well as you did previously. However, your comparison can't be your life prior to the pandemic, just as you can't compare yourself to your peers or to a younger version of yourself. You are who you are at this moment in time—a unique person with experiences that are exclusive to you. Accepting yourself as you are is a choice that can only be made in the present moment.

In short, at any given point in time, regardless of how you feel, you're either doing what gives your life meaning or you're not. Maybe you can't engage in meaningful activities as well as you used to or as much as you'd like. However, *any* movement toward what's truly important to you is movement in the right direction and energy well spent.

Human history is replete with examples of people rising above horrific circumstances to lead exemplary lives. It's a common theme in human existence, so much so that every major religion has a fundamental teaching about the necessity of accepting pain and truth in your life in order to live fully. This is not an accident. What ACT shows us, especially through acceptance, is that no matter what happens in our lives, we are *always* whole. In fact, it's the very experiences that we fear will break us that make us complete as human beings, along with all of the joy and happiness that comes from living life fully.

Julie's Acceptance Story

I absolutely respect medical science. This isn't an abstract appreciation. It's saved my life a few times. It's saved the lives of people I love. Plus, science is cool! And yet, I'm not a fan of doctoring. Certainly you'd think something serious like chest pains would override my kneejerk avoidance. And you'd be right. But I took the scenic route.

It started innocently enough with a burning sensation that progressed into bona fide chest pains that I monitored for a few days (okay, four). They came in intense waves that got closer and closer until I was spending most of my time curled up on the couch hugging a heating pad. It seemed clear that they weren't going to go away on their own. And it was getting harder to tune out my husband's insistence that I see a doctor.

(His appeals came with fun facts like "denial is one of the top symptoms of a heart attack.")

So, I relented and went to an urgent care clinic. Yep, for my *severe chest pains*, I went to a place designed to treat patients with non-life-threatening conditions. (I'd like to tell you this was the first time I went to a clinic for a serious condition, but it's not.) I described my symptoms to the doctor and gave her my interpretation. "I have a chest cold." I maintain that it was pretty creative of me to invent a non-life-threatening condition to go with my urgent care choice.

The doctor checked me out, asked questions, and gave me her assessment. "I fail to see why you think this is a cold. You're having chest pains. You need to go to the ER." I was instantly snapped into reality! No, just kidding. I didn't argue with her, but I was still in denial. The doctor told me again that I had to go to the ER. She explained why. She asked me if I was going to go. Did I have someone to take me? Was I considering it? I answered her with silence, which is very unlike me. She finally looked me in the eye and begged me to go to the ER. "Please, please, please will you? Please tell me you'll go." (I'd like to apologize to her and all of the over-burdened urgent care doctors who have to deal with people like me.)

So, now I know that my avoidant brain can interpret severe chest pains as a cold and I have some extremely creative cognitive dissonance when faced with doctoring. I accept that I have to see my doctors regularly, unpleasant as I think it might be. And when *I notice that I'm having the thought* that I don't want to schedule my follow up appointments, I ask myself if avoidance will keep me from doing things I value. (It might.)

Julie's Tip: My main hurdle in using ACT is remembering to use it, so I like to consciously identify my behavioral cues. For example, I correlate my avoidant coping mechanisms to the threat response: fight, flight, or freeze. Fight is when I'm chatty and full of excuses, which I treat with defusion. Flight is when

I'm distracting myself, which I treat by contacting the present (more on that in Chapter 6). Freeze is when I clam up in denial, which I treat with acceptance.

at this point is another adaption of one of Russ Harris' (2009) designed to help you visualize self-as-context.

Imagine you're a lighthouse keeper on a dark and stormy night. As you cast your light over the sea and the shoreline, you see rocks, waves, and ships. The things illuminated by the beam represent your concept of who you are—the content of your life—healthy or ill, employed or not, happy or sad, calm or distressed. The light itself is your ability to be aware of these things, or self-awareness, if you prefer to think of it that way.

The light is *always emanating from you*. The ships will come and go. The shoreline will erode. The tide will ebb and flow. The weather will be stormy and calm. Regardless of what the light is shining upon, it always comes from the same place—the lighthouse. As the lighthouse operator, you get to choose where the light shines and what gets illuminated. While the content of your life may change dramatically from time to time, maybe even from moment to moment, your awareness of it always comes from you and your choices. We have no control over the ships and the tides and the rocks on the shore, just as you had no control over the COVID-19 virus and its impact on your life.

However, as the lighthouse keeper, you get to point the light wherever you choose for whatever purpose. The lighthouse, therefore, is a safe place from which you can observe the events and content of your life objectively and flexibly. It's difficult to see where the rocks are if you're in a boat on rough seas. But from the lighthouse, this is a much easier task. That's where you want to be, and that's where self-as-context seeks to take you.

Self-Stories: We all tell ourselves stories about who we are. We've done this from the moment we possessed the language and cognitive abilities to do so. (For the record, that's pretty young. It starts to happen very early in childhood.) These stories tend to stick with us, whatever they may be, take your pick— *I'm too fat, no one likes me, I'm not smart enough, I'm unlovable, everyone is better than I am*. They're largely the byproducts of our life experiences, such as getting chosen last for the team, being picked on, experiencing a failure, or even receiving an unintentionally snide comment. However, even if we haven't been traumatized or victimized, we have stories. Some are culturally infused—*I come from a long line of big eaters.* And some even have a favorable spin—*I never get sick, I'm tough, I'm considerate.*

When you tell yourself one of your stories, you've got the beam of light focused intensely on one particular rock along the shore. In other words, you're letting the *content* of your life define your sense of self. When this focus interferes with what you really want to do in your life, you're over-engaging with these old harmful stories and doing yourself a great disservice. Every time you limit yourself because you're living your life according to your stories, you stop yourself from being flexible enough to do things that might be meaningful or beneficial. However, as the lighthouse operator, you can shine the light wherever and whenever you want. In other words, *you* get to decide how much attention gets paid to anything because the light always emanates from you.

Using Self-Stories: While you can simply let your self-stories be without paying them any attention, you can also use them to find your values.

Let's say you're having a hard time coping with these pandemic-related circumstances you didn't plan for. It crosses your mind that it would help to talk to a friend, but you don't want to be a bother. You can tough it out. There are two self-stories here—*I'm a bother* and *I'm tough*—both preventing you from connecting with your friend. But if you adjust the lighthouse beam slightly, you'll see that *I'm a bother* is close to a rocky outcrop that says *I value friendship*. This slightly different perspective can help you remember that reaching out to your friends for moral support and advice isn't bothersome. In fact, it will likely strengthen your bonds. But you're *tough!* Or maybe it's more accurate to say you *value resiliency,* which will come in handy in this instance. You can certainly call on your resiliency to pull you through with the help of a friend.

I'm tough and *I'm a bother* are still there, lying on the shore beyond the light. It's not your job to obliterate them or erase any of the stories of your life. The rocks are part of the shoreline, and the events that created your self-stories are part of who you are. But they don't have to *define* who you are, or more importantly, what you do. *You* get to decide what to pay attention to, what stories matter the most to you, and which ones can help you move forward in a valued direction.

Noticing and Self-Stories: An aspect of self-as-context that can help increase flexibility is the ever-present ACT technique of noticing. To notice what's happening at any given point in time in your life *and in your mind*, ask yourself:

- What's happening right now, in this moment?
- What story is my mind telling me right now?
- Is this story familiar, one of my "Greatest Hits"?
- How does this story go again?
- Does this have to be my truth in this moment?

Even if you don't think you have any negative self-stories, when your life gets turned upside down, things you've always believed about yourself can become roadblocks. Maybe the roles you played in your life never caused you any trouble because you didn't have any conflict. Naturally, you'll blame the pandemic for your situation, rightfully so. But when you notice the stories your circumstances have brought to light, you can decide how to react. For example:

Let's say you never worried about having lots of friends because you've always had them. But after all of the lockdowns, quarantines, and travel bans on top of life changes and shifting priorities, your friendships have changed dramatically. You might think *I'm unlovable.* (You might be able to see that this painful statement shows how much you value friendship.)

Maybe you're sick with long haul symptoms and no one has offered to help despite your willingness to be there for others when you're able. You might say to yourself *I'm always doing for others without reciprocation.* (It's probably safe to say you value helping others and treating them with compassion.)

Or possibly you lost your job doing something you loved in a career you worked hard at for years. You might think *I'm nothing without my work.* (Maybe you value being productive or contributing to your field.)

Even though these painful stories are often evidence of something you value, simply noticing your thoughts can be a powerful tool. It may have seemed like the things you told yourself about who you are were unavoidable facts. But with some distance, you can see them for what they are—stories, not absolute truths. When you remember that, you give yourself the flexibility to shine your spotlight elsewhere.

Apply Self-as-Context to Your Pandemic-Related Circumstances

Self-as-context is an in-the-moment process that requires you to be present in your current life experience—the good, the bad, and the ugly. You might have tried being the person you were before the pandemic—staying in the life you lived because things were better before. But it simply isn't your current reality. Aspects of your life may have been stripped from you—freedom, health, functioning, job, purpose, family role, maybe even your home, family, or friends. Under such dire and extreme circumstances, it's as harmful to attempt to live in your comfortable self-stories from the past as it is to let the dysfunctional ones keep you from living your life right now.

Naturally, being present with painful experiences can be difficult. But self-as-context shows us that we don't have to engage with our stories or make decisions based on them. *You get to choose where to shine the light that will guide the ships where you want them to go.*

Julie's Self-as-Context Story

The last work trip I went on was to Hawaii where I saw two octopuses while I was snorkeling. (Two!) Then I got sick, the country started going into lockdown, and I was laid off. It made logical sense that I couldn't travel anymore. I didn't like this new reality, but it was easy to accept.

Seeing as I was out of breath from walking up a few steps, it wasn't the worst time to be grounded. Sure, losing my sweet travel job was a blow, but I'd find work and ways to travel. However, rebuilding my strength continued to be frustrating because *I'm never going to be able to do the things I used to do!* When I looked closely at this thought, what I was really worried about was how I'd be able to travel in the future. The underlying self-story is that *I have stamina!*

With two athletic older sisters, I'd been muscling through to keep up since I learned how to walk. Difficult hikes, peddling up steep hills, carrying a heavy backpack over cobblestone streets, snorkeling until I was a prune, pounding the pavement of a new city—I've always been able to see what I wanted to see, do what I wanted to do, and push through when I was tired. Until I wasn't. It was a blow to my identity. My stamina was built step by grueling step over a lifetime. First it was based on a comparison to my sisters, then traveling companions, and eventually an old version of myself.

There's certainly nothing wrong with stamina, but I didn't have it anymore. What I was left with was persistence, a mental trait I can have no matter how I change. I'm aware that these words are so similar, they're practically the same. But to me, they're worlds apart. Even when I have no stamina, I can absolutely be persistent as I build up my strength. In fact, it helps if I am.

Julie's Tip: I use a classic trick to help me shift my view. I imagine pinning one of my self-stories on a friend. (*You'll never be able to travel like you used to.*) I'd never think this about a friend or define any of my friends by their circumstances. It's laughable.

Chapter 6

Contact with the Present Moment—Be Here Now

Realize deeply that the present moment is all you ever have. Make the Now the primary focus of your life.
—Eckhart Tolle

Get Centered with Contact with the Present Moment

Contact with the present moment is the second of the "centered" processes essential to developing psychological flexibility. Even though we're all instinctively aware that the present is all we ever have—it's where, when, and how we exist—being in the moment isn't easy for most of us. The good news is that it's a skill anyone can cultivate by getting curious about the here and now.

Allowing yourself to experience each moment fully without judgment or reservation but with self-compassion and openness can have a profound impact on your experience of your life.

Understand Contact with the Present Moment

If the past has already happened and the future has yet to happen, then right now, in this present moment, the past and future are simply constructs of our mind. Unfortunately, they're constructs we tend to pay more attention to than what's happening in the present. As you have no doubt noticed, this inability to remain in contact with the present gets us into trouble and robs us of the moment-to-moment experiences of our lives. In fact, some would argue that it robs us of our lives altogether.

Our minds have a bad habit of dragging us back to the past, revisiting regrets, sorrows, and should-haves. It comes in all shapes and sizes and does us virtually no good whatsoever.

Certainly your past is important. It informs who you are. But learning from your past is a whole lot different from missing your present because you're repeatedly turning it over in your mind, wishing for a different outcome. That's an exercise in futility that we spend an awful lot of time on.

The future holds a similar allure. It kicks our minds into high gear as we try to make sure everything will happen the way we want it to, soothing us with a sense of control. Certainly there are things over which you have a fair degree of control. Chances are pretty good that if you do your job well, you'll keep it. If you maintain your relationships, you'll have a robust social life. If you take care of yourself, you won't get sick. But as we can all attest, these actions don't carry with them any guarantee. You can do everything you possibly can to steer your life in the direction you want it to go, but you may still get blindsided by something like a novel coronavirus. Therefore, attempts to control your future should be undertaken with the greatest of care and with your eyes wide open. Bad things can and do happen, leaving us with a present that we didn't bargain for or expect.

You may be wondering how focusing on a present moment that's painful, heartbreaking, or excruciating can help anything. The answer to this is rather simple—not *easy* but simple. To put it plainly, what choice do you have? Delving into the past won't change anything. You can't go back. Engaging in that process only feeds your suffering. Similarly, overexerting yourself to control your future can be just as futile. Your future can't impact your current circumstances, which is what you're experiencing *at this very moment* in your life. So, again, what choice do you have but to stay present?

If you're like most people and have a hard time staying present, you can blame your big problem-solving brain, luring you to troubleshoot your past and future problems. (*Thanks, mind!*) The good news is that you don't have to possess any particular talent or innate ability in order to stay present. In fact, active mindfulness can be practiced anywhere, anytime, while you're doing almost anything. As long as there's a present moment at hand, and there always is, there's an opportunity to be mindful of it—when you're washing the dishes, taking a walk, eating a meal. Whatever the moment brings, the idea is to be present with that, even if it's painful or difficult.

Being completely and totally focused on what's happening right now takes practice and patience. It's not easy, but when you start really working at this, your skill and your life will improve.

Active Mindfulness is simply awareness during your daily activities. When someone says "mind your manners," "mind your step," or "mind the gap" in London, they're politely saying "pay attention." If you're mindful while you do the dishes, you're fully focusing on them and nothing else. It's easier to connect with focused awareness if you think of a hobby. Let's say you enjoy gardening or playing tennis or painting. You're not picking tomatoes, serving the ball, or adding happy little trees while you're going over your list of things to do, agonizing about a social faux pas, or worrying about your future. You're concentrating on the task at hand. And this is an enjoyable experience. It might even be utterly absorbing. Likewise, if we harness our attention to focus on everyday activities, it can bring similar pleasures to mundane tasks. This is, in essence, a form of experiential acceptance in the present moment. Additionally, when you focus your attention, you build this invaluable skill, the same one your self-as-context uses to concentrate on things that matter most to you. Next time you face a sink full of dishes, try it. Mind the sponge.

Practice Noticing: Being mindful and present is all about paying exquisite attention to—or noticing—the present moment. It may be your thoughts, physical sensations, emotions, the food you're eating, the flower you're smelling, or the conversation you're having—it doesn't matter. All that matters is that you're attending to it and nothing else.

It's perfectly normal to lose your focus on the present moment. It's an exceedingly rare individual who can be fully present all of the time. So be gentle with yourself as you develop this skill. Stop, breathe, and take a moment to focus on that breath. When you catch yourself drifting, treat yourself with compassion and keep coming back to the present. As you keep redirecting and practicing, you'll eventually find you're redirecting less and less while you're existing in the present moment more and more.

Use Anchors: Anchors can help ground you in the present moment, stopping your mind from pulling you into the past or future. They can be anything that gets you focused on your present experience. You've likely experienced mindfulness when deeply immersed in something you truly enjoy— taking a walk in nature, participating in sports, indulging in a hobby, being with family, reading a great book, eating a favorite food. Any pleasurable activity can cause spontaneous mindfulness. If you pay attention to these moments, you can find the anchors that work best for you.

- **Sensations**: Our sensory experience is an ever-present anchor that always exists in the moment. At any time we can return to the present by focusing on what we see, hear, smell, feel, or taste. For example, paying attention to your breath is a common way to quickly bring your awareness to three of your senses at once. As you feel, smell, and hear the air going into and out of your lungs, you're pulled away from your worries and into the present.
- **Activities**: If you have a hobby that you focus on so

intently that everything else falls away, this is an anchor. You can't always indulge in your hobbies, but you can notice the mindfulness skill they've given you and carry it through to other areas of your life. For example, activities that have a rote element to them like kayaking or knitting or running, can be harnessed for other areas of your life. Simply identifying your ability to tolerate repetition and persist can help you improve your endurance with tasks you find boring.

- **Values**: When you connect your present to what's important to you, it creates richly meaningful moments you're less likely to be pulled away from. For example, let's say right now in the present moment, you're avoiding getting on the treadmill. Sure, your health is important to you, but it's not the thing that drives you. So, ask yourself, what *do* you live for? Let's say your kids are the most important things in your life. You value being a good parent. If you connect your present struggle with your drive to be a good parent, it's easier to take action. Now when you get on the treadmill, you're setting a healthy example for your kids and building endurance so you can enjoy more activities with them.

- **People**: Just like your values make the present moment rich and meaningful, so do the people you love, who you naturally focus on with exquisite attention. Even if you're a bit of a lone wolf, all humans are inherently social beings. We're hardwired to make meaningful connections with others. And the bonds we have with each other are deeply rewarding. Just like immersion in our hobbies can give us residual benefits for mundane tasks, the skills we have from deeply focusing on our loved ones can be carried over into other areas of our lives.

Practice Contact with the Present Moment

There is something about leaning into your present moment experience—choosing not to fight it, run away from it, or change it, but just embracing it fully for what it is by observing it, noticing it, and letting it be—that fundamentally transforms the quality of your experience of that present. It won't absolve you from emotional pain or difficulty, but it can change how you experience it in your life. This is the goal. Remember, ACT is not designed to help you feel *differently*, it is designed to help you *feel* differently. Noticing and embracing your present is a big step in this direction.

Explore Your Senses Mindfully: Following is a basic mindfulness exercise to help you focus on your sensory experiences. You might want to record yourself (or someone else) to guide you through the exercise. If you find yourself wandering, as everyone does, gently acknowledge that you stepped outside of the moment and bring yourself back. "Coming back to center" is an invaluable skill you can develop, so know that every time you do it, you're getting better at it.

Settle yourself comfortably in a quiet place where you won't be interrupted. Close your eyes or keep them fixed on a specific point on the floor or the wall. Take a few nice, easy breaths. As you breathe in, focus on how the cool air feels in your nose and mouth, moving down your windpipe and into your lungs. As you breathe out, focus on how the warm, air feels leaving your body. Continue to focus on your breathing for a little bit. Now turn your attention to the rest of your senses. Focus on how the seat feels against your legs, your back, your arms... how your hands feel in your lap or at your sides. Focus on any sounds you might be able to hear, the heater or air conditioner blowing in the room, traffic or wind outside, the house settling. Welcome the experience of the sound and focus on how it feels... the sound moving into your ear. On your next breath in, notice if there are any smells in the air, and breathe them in. Focus on the quality of the smell. Is it bitter or sweet, pleasant or unpleasant? Do you taste anything as you breathe in? Breathe it in and let it become part of you. Now pay attention to your total sensory experience—everything you feel, smell, hear, and taste. Allow those sensations to be there and focus on them. If you drift off and your mind wanders, that's okay. Gently acknowledge it and bring your full attention back to your sensory experience. Now, take a moment to return to the focus on your breath, the coolness on the in-breath, the warmth of the out-breath. Focus on that for a bit… and open your eyes when you feel ready and comfortable.

Doing this exercise with any degree of regularity will serve as a great foundation for being mindful in difficult and triggering circumstances.

Be a Detective and a Documentarian: Rather than sink into worry or frustration, you can use your emotions as reminders to contact the present moment. If you find yourself worrying, this is a cue to be the detective. Get out your magnifying glass and turn your attention to what you see right now. Look at what is, not what could be or what was. If you find yourself frustrated by your pain and discomfort, this is a great time to become your own documentary filmmaker—put yourself behind the video camera and focus on the broader context of your life. Here's how:

- **The Detective**: To pull out of worry and return to the present, pretend you're Sherlock Holmes, noticing every detail in the moment, intently focused on your environment. Zero in on the present moment, whether it's listening to a friend, noticing how the air feels going into your lungs, or tasting a sip of water. Simply be in the moment. Put each detail under the magnifying glass and observe what you're experiencing without judgment openly and freely.

- **The Documentarian**: When the details of your present experience are overwhelming or frustrating, pull back and take a broader view. As the director of your own documentary, you can point the camera anywhere you like. Sweep the landscape taking in all of the colors. Track the crowded highway. Pan the waiting room at the doctor's office. Scout the location and notice any interesting features. Zoom in on a face or the texture of a fabric then pull back and capture a conversation. Like any good documentarian, point the camera at the action whenever possible. If you're talking with friends, focus on what they're saying, the words they choose, their vocal quality, and body language. And if you're alone, notice your room, your body in repose, or a beam of light coming through the window.

  It is important to note that the documentarian view isn't about trying to distance yourself from your pain, be it physical or emotional. That would be akin to avoidance. However, your pain is only part of the larger picture of your experience and your life. Yes, it's present and you do experience it, but you also experience love, joy, friendship, and any activity you're able to engage in. The video camera allows you to place your current experience of the moment in a broader context.

Being able to move back and forth between the focused and broad perspectives can be hugely powerful in helping you stay present. It gives you ways to experience whatever life is giving you *at* that moment *in* that moment, rather than trying to avoid or move away from it. When you start doing this, you'll soon see that your experience encompasses so much more than your pain.

Apply Contact with the Present Moment to Your Pandemic Pain

Embracing your present and being mindful doesn't mean we reject, ignore, or abandon the past or the future. Paying attention to these aspects of our lives is important to our survival, which is why we have this amazing skill. But over attending to them can be simply disastrous. Your mind will try to drag you down that rabbit hole on a nearly continuous basis to no useful end. Additionally, distracting ourselves from a present that has moments of pain, loss, or hopelessness doesn't work. It doesn't make the pain or loss go away, and it doesn't move us toward the things we value. Mindful attention to the present is the antidote.

There's a mountain of scientific literature that shows the profound impact mindfulness can have on your functioning and your experience of your life. However, it takes effort to experience your present flexibly and without judgment or reservation. It's something that ultimately you'll experience as a series of failures until you realize that the only thing you ever need to do is recognize when you drift, forgive yourself, and redirect your attention to the moment. Notice and come back, notice and come back, and keep going as best you can.

Julie's Contact with the Present Moment Story

I love being in the present moment—close ups, long views, conversations, hikes, travels, writing, editing, reading, eating, playing with my pets. However, my natural state is to be in my head. So I'm still not great at being mindful despite having cultivated this skill for over three decades. (In fact, it was Joe who introduced me to it with a meditation exercise when we were in high school.)

Sometimes being present is easy. My sister likes to tell this story about when the moving truck we were driving 300 miles from our grandmother's broke down halfway to our dad's. My sister called the rental company, and I unwrapped the lunch, with my favorite sandwich, that our grandmother packed us. We ate in silence while we waited on the side of the road. My sister was worrying about what we were going to do, how long it would take, would someone be able to fix the truck, would we have to load everything into a new truck? She looked over at me to commiserate and found me gazing at my food. "What are you thinking about?" she asked. I looked over at her then back. "I was just wondering which bite of this sandwich I should take next." The rental company fixed the truck in a minute, and she still teases me for not worrying about it. Of course, I can't always eat my favorite sandwich instead of pointlessly worrying.

Sometimes being present isn't easy but it's the best option available. When I'm in physical pain and my brain isn't working so well, I'll reach for the low hanging fruit of my visual experience. For example, in the hospital getting a cardiac catheter jammed into my tender arm, there was no point in focusing on that kind of pain. It wouldn't be useful (unlike the information about my chest pain—quality, intensity, duration, change—which was useful to my doctors). So, after I indicated that the catheter hurt (just in case they were doing it wrong), I shifted my attention to the broad view, dialing into the hulking plastic-covered medical equipment that was lurching around me. And now I know how to make a convincing alien abduction video. (Useful!)

Sometimes being present is impossible. I still like to daydream and imagine and ruminate. And I'll completely forget that being in the moment is even an option when I've got an agenda. For example, when I was ready to leave the hospital I was so intent on getting released that I forced conversations with anyone who would listen to go in that direction—doctors, nurses, the woman who was just trying to take out the trash. I definitely missed some opportunities to talk about my care. (Oops.)

Julie's Tip: While I've used the close-up and broad views

Chapter 7

Values—What Matters Most

You rarely have time for everything you want in this life, so you need to make choices. And hopefully, your choices can come from a deep sense of who you are.
—**Fred Rogers**

Engage with Values

For the last several chapters, you've probably gathered that it's not in our best interest to make decisions about our behaviors and our lives based on stories our minds tell us, emotional experiences we want to chase or avoid, outdated versions of ourselves, or moments in which we've gotten stuck. Assuming you're on board with all of this to some degree, it begs a very important question. *If we're not making decisions based on our thoughts, feelings, perspective of self, the past, or the future, then how do we know what to do in any given situation?*

The answer to this is as clear as anything could ever be in the ACT model. It's something you've probably heard a thousand times before in a thousand different places from a thousand different people—your parents, teachers, friends, relatives, coaches, or even therapists. We need to make decisions, all of our decisions, based on our values. This may be a loaded term for many people. It tends to conjure up notions of religion, morality, ethics, or laws—all of which may be related to your values but aren't necessarily. Values from an ACT perspective are yours and yours alone. Values work can be the best part of life and one of the most invigorating aspects of ACT. Once you identify your values—*what you live for, your principles, what's important in your life*—they will be the touchstones that help you see how life is full of experiences you can apply meaning to.

From there, very little can stop you.

Values, your principles that reflect what's important in your life, are constant and are never really achieved. They are ever-present in our lives and are the criteria upon which we base all of our decisions. You're never "done" having values.

Understand Values

It is not the intention of this chapter, this book, or ACT for that matter to define your values for you. While the word may carry with it a variety of connotations for you, some good, maybe some not so good, it's important that you understand exactly how ACT defines and uses values to help you live a better life. From an academic perspective, Wilson and Dufrene (2010) describe values in the following way: "In ACT, values are freely chosen, verbally constructed consequences of ongoing, dynamic, evolving patterns of activity, which establish predominant reinforcers for that activity that are intrinsic in engagement in the valued behavioral pattern in itself." This is a mouthful, but let's take a closer look and see what they're really saying and what that means for you.

Values Are Freely Chosen: The fact that your values are freely chosen is fantastic news. It means that this is one of the few areas in your life where *you have complete and total control.* Assuming your values don't involve anything that advocates directly hurting others, such as abuse or assault, no ACT therapist or ACT book is going to tell you what you should or should not value. While you may not be able to control your mind or your emotions, you do get to control your values. This is a primary difference between ACT and many other imposed value systems whether they're from religions, parents, or peers. While any of those groups may play important roles in how you decide what your values are, ultimately, *you* decide what they are—what matters to you, what's meaningful, and what direction you want your life to take.

The flip side to this is that freely choosing your values can be overwhelming. Many of us go through life so caught up in our pain or our attempts to avoid pain that we're completely disconnected from our own values. This contributes to a downward spiral in life and can lead to profound suffering. Ironically, when faced with the prospect of freely choosing one's values, people often freeze up, become paralyzed, or avoid the process altogether. Another reason for this is that our values are often intimately connected to our pain, which gets the experiential avoidance train running at full speed.

Values Are Action Based: As you know, ACT is deeply rooted in behavioral principles, and values are no different in the ACT model. While we can certainly have feelings-based values, such as valuing the love of your family, ACT is far more focused on action-based values. In other words, what do you *do* to move closer to what's vital, meaningful, and deeply important in your life? Ultimately, ACT is about helping you develop psychological flexibility so you can lead a rich, vital, and meaningful life regardless of what pain you may be experiencing. In order for that to happen, you have to be engaged and action oriented. In short, no one gets what they really want out of life by having it drop in their lap. Meaningful lives come about as a result of action, and decisions about those actions need to be based on your values if you're to stay the course. Values serve as the guideposts for our decision-making processes. No matter how cloudy or murky our path may be, those guideposts will always bring us home.

It's not uncommon for people who are in pain to start their values work with "Dead Man's Goals" (Russ Harris, 2009). These are goals or values that a dead person could accomplish better than we could. "I don't want to feel this way anymore" or "I want to stop doing" whatever behavior we've identified as problematic. Because these things are phrased in a negative context, they describe inaction rather than action. The focus is on *not* doing something rather than moving towards something inherently meaningful. Values should always be phrased in the positive. Think of them as guidelines for behavior that you can always move towards. Dead people are really good at *not* feeling things and *not* doing things. We need to be the opposite.

This is particularly relevant if you're suffering. You're very likely to think about your life and your values in terms of what you don't want. You don't want to be tired. You don't want to be in pain. You don't want to be grieving. You don't want to be unemployed. This is a natural response, but it has no place in determining your values because values have to be something you can move towards. Focusing on what you don't want will only contribute to you continuing to feel stuck. Framing your values as something to act on offers the potential for meaningful change.

Values Are Intrinsic: Engaging in values-based behavior is intrinsically rewarding. What that means is the value is in the behavior itself, not because it might bring some additional benefit. Sometimes an additional benefit comes anyway, and it's great when this happens, but the behavior is its own reward. This can be a difficult concept for people to grasp. For example, a lot of us work because we need to make money to pay the bills. But some of us work because we love the work we do. Sure, we get paid too, but the real reward is in the work itself, even if it's simply the value of doing something versus being unproductive. What really matters is the work, not so much the money.

I ask every client I see what's truly important to them, what matters most in their lives, and I do it the very first time I meet them. Very few people tell me they want to be rich and powerful. Most tell me things like they want to be healthy, be a good parent, a good spouse, or make a positive mark on the world. These are all intrinsic values; they provide internal satisfactions. In other words, they are rewarding in and of themselves. So ask yourself this question as a starting point and remain open to further clarifying your values.

Values Are Not Goals: People often confuse goals with values, but there's a simple way to tell the difference. If it has a clear end point, it's a goal. For example, graduating from college, having a job, or being a parent are all goals because they are achievable. However, don't throw away your goals. They are valuable signposts as they're often and ideally supported by and grounded in values, which are constant and never really achieved. They are ever-present in our lives and are the criteria upon which we base all of our decisions. You're never done having values.

For example, if I want to be a father, that's a goal, not a value. Once I have children, that goal is achieved and it no longer guides my decision-making process. However, if I want to be a good father, that's a value. It's something that I will never be done working towards (hopefully). Almost every decision I make in my life is infused with this value. If I think of the characteristics of being a good father—being present, expressing love and support, providing for my family, being a good husband to my wife, serving as a model for the kind of person I would want my children to marry—all of these things guide me in my decision-making processes, including how I interact with my children, what I do with my time, how I treat my wife, whether I volunteer at my daughters' schools, and so forth. I am never "done" being a good father.

Similarly, the values you identify can never be achieved or completed. If you think about the things that are important to you in the various domains of your life—work, family, health, leisure, spirituality—the values you connect to those things should be ever-present and serve as guideposts. They will always keep you on course.

Values Are Big Picture and Unifying: When asked to identify our values, we often respond with things we'd like to do or be. "I value my work" or "I value being a parent" might be some common answers to what you value. As discussed earlier, values are action-oriented, but they should be identified with the quality of the action, not the action itself. While it's fine to value work or being a parent, it's more meaningful to identify the quality of how one works or is a parent.

For example, I value my work as a psychologist and a teacher, but there are qualities to that work that I identify as particularly valuable. Each provides an important service to others that hopefully enhances the quality and meaning of their lives. Both are intellectually stimulating and challenging and allow me to meet interesting people from whom I can learn (and teach) new things on a regular basis. It's these underlying qualities of my jobs that represent the real values of my work. It is also important to note that these things do not have to be specific to my work. I can learn new things, meet new people, and enhance the lives of others in a variety of ways and situations.

If you have been robbed of the ability to engage in activities you love, identifying your values is absolutely critical. For example, maybe you are one of the many people whose activity level has been drastically reduced by your COVID infection. You likely are struggling with your inability to engage in valued activities, and rightfully so. However, if you dig deeper into the values "treasure chest" and look at the issue more globally, you might see that while the specific activity may have been enjoyable, it was enjoyable because it connected you to something you valued—maybe it was being close to nature, getting away from the hustle and bustle of day-to-day life, or doing an activity with someone you care about and being connected to that person in a specific way.

I love to climb mountains with my best friend from childhood. Probably 70 percent of the reason I do that activity is to bond with my friend. The activity is simply a vehicle for me to get to do what I really value—connect to another human being by sharing unique life experiences. At some point, we won't climb mountains anymore, whether it's because we're just no longer physically able or, as our wives would say, we've finally come to our senses. However, even though that activity won't be available to us, we can still connect with each other and make decisions that move us towards that value not away from it. And that's what matters.

Typically, there comes a time in our lives when we can't do what we love as well as we used to. Athletes lose the physical ability to compete like they used to as they get older. Musicians can't play their instruments the same way they did when they were 25, or maybe they can't play at all anymore because of illness or injury. COVID may have brought you to this point earlier than you wanted, but that time when we "can't" anymore always comes earlier than we want it to. So what do you do? When you realize that the love of the sport drives the athlete and the love of music drives the musician, you find other ways to engage with that love. Or maybe the athlete's value is in being competitive. If so, then the game may change but the satisfaction remains. The musician could simply enjoy being expressive or creative, which can be accomplished in so many fulfilling new ways. You coach, you teach, you write, you watch, you listen. You do anything you can to stay connected to what is ultimately the larger value. Vehicles that move us towards our values can change even if the value itself doesn't. You may not be able to drive the fancy sports car anymore, but you can still drive something—even an old clunker can get you where you need to be. The idea is to stay engaged with your values in any way you can.

Whatever has been taken from you, find out what it was about it that really mattered to you. If you loved your work that you can't do anymore, ask yourself why you loved your work? What was it about the job or the career that you really valued? Was it that you were accomplishing something? Did you enjoy being in charge? Helping others? Providing for your family? How else can you do that in a way that's possible for you now? The answers may not be perfect or "as good as before," but that comparison isn't a worthwhile thought to be engaging in. It's simply your mind trying to spoil your party and keep you from being in the moment and engaged with what matters most in your life.

Values can *never* be taken away from you by anything or anyone. COVID may have robbed you of the vehicle through which you used to engage with your values, but it cannot rob you of your values themselves—nothing can. No matter what has happened to you in your life, you can always make choices to engage in a values-driven life. It might not be pain free, as Viktor Frankl knew all too well, but moving away from your values will only prolong and increase your suffering.

Find Your Values

Values work can be satisfying, fun, and also difficult, particularly if you've spent your life chasing emotional satisfaction and avoiding pain. Thankfully, the ACT folks have done a lot of work creating exercises that will help you to construct your value system—and it *is* a matter of construction. Your values are all yours. You have complete and total control, which doesn't happen often. Enjoy!

As with most of the ACT exercises in this book, these techniques are presented in other works as well. The ones listed below are taken or adapted from a list created by Russ Harris (2009) who has done amazing work in making ACT accessible to everyone. I encourage you to avail yourself of these additional resources. The exercises below are designed to help you construct your values. I don't expect that all of these will resonate with you (nor should you), but I do suspect that some of them will. You won't know which ones will do the trick for you until you try them.

Speeches: Imagine yourself at an event that's being given in your honor. Listen to the speeches the important people in your life give about you—how their lives have been affected by you, what you stand for, and what you mean to them. If you've lived your life as the person you want to be, what do you imagine these people saying?

Role Models: Think of someone you admire—a friend, family member, historical figure, leader, innovator—anyone really. What are their strengths? What do you admire about them? Now imagine you've lived your life like them. What would you need to do to become more like this image you have of yourself?

Wealth: You've hit the lottery! With all financial barriers removed, you're free to do whatever you want. What will it be? With whom do you share the money, time, and experiences your newfound wealth has given you?

Magic Wand: With the wave of a magic wand, everything you do is met with full approval. No matter what you do, you're universally liked and respected, whether you're a philanthropist or a hermit. What do you do with your life? How do you treat others? With another wave of the wand, all painful thoughts, feelings, and memories cease to affect you. How does your life change? What do you do more of? Less of?

The Sweet Spot: As vividly as possible, recall a moment in your life that was sweet or touching. What was it about this event that was so meaningful? How is that connected to your values and what's important to you?

Disapproval: We can learn a lot from the things we don't like, especially in the actions of others. Perhaps you don't tolerate rudeness, dishonesty, or laziness. Knowing what you don't appreciate can lead to important insights into what really matters to you and how you want to conduct your life.

Missing Out: Is there anything in your life that you're holding back from doing? Are there things that you'd like to do but aren't doing because you're avoiding some painful aspect of that activity? Is there something you'd like to do but are avoiding because you're worried about the future? What are you missing out on because of fear?

Your Pain: Dig through the wasteland of your difficult memories for the buried treasure within. Values and pain go hand in hand. If you're having difficulty identifying what matters to you most, look to your pain (and your avoidance of pain). It's a fundamental principle of ACT that we can't lead a values-driven life without also experiencing pain. Additionally, right now you are likely in a good degree of pain. Use it.

How Values Work Works: Let's say you've always been social—volunteering, throwing parties, and eating out with friends. The pandemic has changed all of this, causing you pain. Pain is a cue to explore your values. In this case, you'd ask yourself what it is that you love about being social. If you say you value friendship, but video chatting with a group of friends isn't fulfilling your needs, you might need to dig deeper and look at the specific activities to find the values they reflect:

- Why do I like volunteering? *It makes me feel good to **contribute positively** to making the world a better place.*
- Why do I enjoy throwing neighborhood parties? *It's **fun**!*
- Why do I eat out with friends? *I like **connecting authentically** with my inner circle.*

With your values clarified—contributing positively, having fun, connecting authentically—you can now find ways to engage with them in different ways. You could volunteer virtually, play a game online with your neighbors, and call a close friend to have a genuine conversation. When you identify and connect your actions to your values, the satisfaction remains even when the activities change. Your pandemic-related limits might make it harder, even impossible, for you to engage in your values in ways that are comfortable and familiar to you, but there are always alternatives. The new activities might not be as enjoyable, but that comparison isn't worthwhile. Defuse from it and stay in the moment. No matter how small an action might be, moving towards your values will always be better than beating yourself up about how much you've lost or can no longer do.

Apply Values with Pandemic Pain

Nothing can strip you of your values—not a pandemic, COVID-19, change, or anything else. They are the grounding forces that give life meaning. Your ability to act may be reduced, but your values remain as large and as important as ever. Additionally, you can defuse more easily from unhelpful thoughts if it leads you toward your values. You can more willingly accept painful emotions and events if they're in service of what you hold dear. And if you get mired in regrets or worries, your values can bring you back to the present and guide you from moment to moment and day to day. Once you're clear on your values, you can always make choices to live a values-driven life.

However, even if we're well connected to what's important to us, sometimes we have to choose one value over another. This is particularly true when life deals us a bum hand. This is an unfortunate reality of life, but it highlights two important aspects of values identification.

First, it's not a bad idea to have a rough sense of how your values are prioritized. You value things in various areas of your life, but some are undoubtedly more important than others. Having a sense of where those priorities are will help you when you're faced with conflicts and difficult decisions.

Second, values are to be used as guides not rules. Sometimes we're simply not able to make decisions or engage in actions that move us towards our values. Beating ourselves up over this serves no purpose whatsoever. While we need to hold on to our values, we shouldn't crush them in our fists. We need to be compassionate and forgiving with ourselves when, on occasion, we don't make the "right" decision or fall down in our efforts to lead values-driven lives. Values are supposed to free us and guide us, not crush us under the weight of unrealistic internal expectations. We do what we can when we can do it, recognize as best as we can when we aren't, and gently redirect ourselves back on the values-driven path. ACT (and life) can be a whole lot easier when you practice this kind of self-compassion.

Julie's Values Story

One of my most vivid childhood memories is from a trip through the US south in the '70s. I saw Spanish moss for the first time! My mom bought a bag of the most delicious oranges I'd ever eaten through the window of the family station wagon! A gargantuan black beetle in our motel room stood its ground as my sisters and I screamed and ran! My young life had never been so exciting.

Travel still gives me a thrill. It fulfills a lot of my psychological needs and is aligned with my top values, including curiosity and novelty. I like discovering new things, problem-solving on the fly, and meeting strangers from a strange land. As you might expect, work travel wasn't always a magical experience. Sometime it was just traffic, box stores, corporate parks, cookie cutter hotels, and small talk. But there was also the full solar eclipse in Kentucky, swimming with wild manatees in Florida, and a massive cloud of bats at dusk in Austin. There's no adequate substitute for this. I can absolutely indulge my curiosity and seek out new experiences in other ways, but nothing else fires on all cylinders. So, when I can't travel, all I can do is take care of myself so I can get the most out of it when I'm able to go again, in whatever way that's possible.

Julie's Tip: It took some time for me to identify my top value, the one I prioritize first. For me, autonomy is so important and integrated into my life, I didn't see it immediately. Forest for the trees, I guess. All of my values in every area of my life live in

Autonomy Forest. It informs my work, relationship, friendships, interactions, health, leisure activities, and deeply held beliefs. In fact, I probably connect so strongly with ACT because it encourages autonomy. Because my life has been designed through the autonomy filter, I don't have a lot of struggles in that area. However, my frustrations and the limititations of the pandemic brought it into sharp focus. And I'm glad for that. It's made my decisions moving forward much easier. As such, I can't recommend more strongly that you stay curious about your values. Keep checking in with yourself. And maybe don't get a tattoo of them right away.

Chapter 8

Committed Action—Doing Is Living

Any action is often better than no action, especially if you have been stuck in an unhappy situation for a long time. If it is a mistake, at least you learn something, in which case it's no longer a mistake. If you remain stuck, you learn nothing.
—Eckhart Tolle

Engage with Committed Action

Committed Action—the "C" in ACT—is where the rubber meets the road. Action is so critically important to ACT, the very acronym reinforces its necessity. Without doing, nothing happens. You remain stuck, unable to move forward and often repeating the same old patterns. However, you also can't simply act, doing the same things over and over in violation of your values. Values without action are useless, and actions without values are directionless at best, destructive at worst.

With values-based actions and decisions, every present moment has a higher purpose and each choice develops a pattern that supports what matters to you.

Understand Committed Action

While you may not have much, if any, control over your own thoughts or feelings, essentially you have total control over your own behavior. You get to choose your actions. Of course, this doesn't mean that you get to do whatever you want whenever you want. There are situations when you simply can't act in the way you want, like when you're limited in any way—physically, mentally, or practically. However, that doesn't mean you can't act in *some* way that moves you closer to what you value. This is a powerful distinction that gives you a much broader range of options—and that range can make all of the difference in your quality of life.

Acknowledging that you choose your actions can ultimately be liberating, but we often experience choice as a burden. We fear that we might make "bad" or "wrong" choices versus "good" or "right" choices. However, in ACT, we sidestep this problem altogether by not focusing on the moralistic aspect of choice. Instead, we focus solely on function. Every action is either "useful" or "not useful" to leading your values-driven life.

Is It Useful? Let go of the weight of good/bad/right/wrong choices by simply thinking of every choice as useful or not. To know if a choice is useful, all you have to do is evaluate it by whether or not it supports your values.

To fully embrace committed action, we first have to tackle the myth of motivation. We're culturally inundated with dysfunctional messages about a mysterious force that drives some of us and not others. Any day of the week you can find seemingly inspirational stories about exceptional individuals who do exceptional things. The hidden message is that these people were incredibly motivated and you have to be too if you want to do anything important or useful. However, it's a myth that motivation has to come *before* the behavior. More often than not, it's *behavior* that facilitates motivation.

People who have accomplished great things—or anything at all—will tell you that they usually weren't feeling particularly motivated when they were training for a marathon, doing their physical therapy, learning a new language, studying hard to pass qualifying exams, or getting lunches made for the kids before they left for school. These people simply decided to act in a way that moved them toward their values. The reinforcing good feelings about doing what was "right" for them, and the resulting motivation, didn't come until *after* the action.

The myth of motivation leads to a subversive trap. You feel like you can't do anything until you're motivated, but as we know, motivation is elusive. Your brain is smart and overprotective of you—it will direct your body to rest and conserve energy as much as possible. It steers you away from hard work that it doesn't deem necessary for immediate survival. The mind convinces you that action is too hard and it's best to just stay put. Sure, once in a while you feel the urge to take action, but if we only took action when we felt like it, we would all be perpetually stuck.

The escape from the elusive trap of the motivation myth is to stop paying attention to how motivated you are, connect your actions with your values, and act accordingly. Notice that second part—*connect your actions with your values*. This is the other piece of the puzzle that most people miss. We tend to act or not act based on how we feel rather than on what's really important to us. If you remember that everything you do is enriching your life in some way, you can quiet the mind chatter—be it fear, entropy, or self-destructive self-talk—that sabotages action. We forget that we're doing something because it's actually important to us on a deeply personal and meaningful level. Thoughts and emotions can be loud, annoying, and interfering, but it's up to you if they determine your actions or not.

A big reason people stay stuck is simply avoidance of pain, be it emotional or physical. This is our natural inclination, and no one should be judged for it—not you or anyone else. However, inaction for the purpose of avoiding pain is not an effective way to live our lives. Committed action can cause discomfort—it probably will at some point—because our values and our pain are intimately connected. You often can't get to one without going through the other. This is why we must remain open to experiencing pain or discomfort *in service of our values*.

Ironically, at some point if you keep acting in your valued direction despite how motivated you may or may not be, the motivation eventually comes. Anyone who has exercised on a regular basis knows that the first couple of months are just brutal. But after a while, you start to look forward to your workouts, and it gets a little bit easier. Not all of the time, but more so than it was before. So, action actually facilitates motivation (not the other way around). It's a cruel irony. But once you open up to action regardless of motivation, it's a powerful skill and will lead to an enriched life.

If we allow our fear of pain to dictate our actions, we are essentially adrift, which in and of itself is painful. Pain that is borne of avoidance quickly turns to suffering. Once you decide to move, to take action toward a valued direction, *that* pain or discomfort has a purpose—and purpose can make all the difference. Sure, occasionally our values-based actions are flat out easy, even fun. When this happens, ride that wave! Open yourself up to it and enjoy.

Practice Committed Action

We've all engaged in that mental back and forth, arguing with ourselves over what to do. If you really listen to what your mind is saying in these moments, you can identify common barriers and release yourself from the paralysis of inaction.

Self-Stories: You probably know the stories you tell yourself. They're usually some version of "the same old story," your "Greatest Hits." *It's too hard. I can do it later. I'm not good enough. I'll fail.* This is your inherently lazy mind trying to trick you into non-action. If you can notice this process and recognize the story, you can defuse from it and increase your chances of taking values-directed action.

Undefined Values: If you're unclear on your values, it'll be difficult to take committed action. You may also have a values conflict or prioritization problems. You might be focusing on goals or rules. Or maybe your values have changed. Take some time to evaluate and get in touch with your values. Once you do, committed action will come easier.

Going Too Big: It's a rare occasion when we bite off more than we can chew and find that meal nourishing. A wise strategy in taking committed action is to make those actions small, realistic, and achievable. If you have grand plans that are overwhelming you into inaction, remember that even the smallest valued action can be powerful.

Waiting for the Perfect Time: In ACT, and in life, you bear the responsibility for your action and your inaction. What we don't do defines us as much as what we do. However, it's through doing that we truly live. If you're stalled, it's within your control to change. Everything doesn't have to be just right before we act. If you willingly embrace doubt and discomfort, you can move forward with whatever actions you deem *useful* to take.

Making Goals the Goal: Because goals are future-based and dependent on achievement, they can rob you of happiness, satisfaction, or contentment in the present. Let's say you're doing everything you can to reach a goal to get healthy. If there's a day you don't reach that goal, you risk disappointment, shame, and guilt. Instead, let's say you value your health. Now with the same actions, you can experience satisfaction regularly whenever you do anything for your health. As a whole series of smaller value driven behaviors, you increase the likelihood of becoming healthier, but pass on the negative self-judgment.

Apply Committed Action Now

In light of the limits and pressures the pandemic has put on you, there's no action too small. And sometimes inaction is the best action of all. ACT is all about embracing the present moment flexibly and fluidly, free of judgment or reproach. It is in this space where we make all of our decisions and experience our lives. Connecting your actions to your values can have a powerful impact on your day-to-day, even moment-to-moment, existence. Every time you act in accordance with your values, you get to live meaningfully right now.

The bottom line is that as long as you're connected with your values and acting in a way that moves you toward them, you're doing okay. You can always make choices that move you toward your values. If you're consistent in this approach, your life will have more meaning than it otherwise would. Will you have the life you envisioned for yourself, the life that you planned for and counted on? Maybe not. But focusing on what you've lost rather than what you have won't lead to any kind of meaningful existence for you or those you love. In whatever way you can, no matter how small, *engage, engage, engage*.

Julie's Committed Action Story

This book is the result of committed action. After months out of work with low energy and my heart health to manage, I missed being useful (something I value). I proposed this project to Joe, who agreed to it despite his ridiculously busy schedule. (He also values helping people in useful ways.)

Editing this book is an example of completely enjoyable values-based action. ACT resonates with me and the information was written by someone I respect wholeheartedly for people who are suffering in ways I can relate to. I'd look at the clock and an hour or two or five would have passed in the blink of an eye.

And then my husband injured his knee badly, severely restricting his mobility. Suddenly, the passing time mattered and my limited energy was needed elsewhere. I had to help him navigate his days and drive him to appointments while handling all of the household chores. I absolutely value my relationship with my husband and would do anything for him, but caretaking isn't my strength.

If I'd been in the middle of a project that wasn't so strongly connected to my values, it would have been difficult to find the time. As it happened, I used the delays to notice my own experiences with ACT. Sure, I would have preferred really sinking in to my work without interruption, but then I wouldn't have this perfect illustration of the merits of values-driven action in the face of competing priorities. I hope you find it useful.

Julie's Tip: If I value being useful in practical ways, caretaking should be a cinch, right? As it turns out, being useful is a value I have around work. In my relationship, I value openness and teamwork. I might not have clarified this if I hadn't had to take care of my husband. So, if you also compartmentalize, take a look at what you value in different areas of your life.

Chapter 9

Bring It All Together—ACT is Fluid and Flexible

All is connected... no one thing can change by itself.
—**Paul Hawken**

Open Up, Center Yourself, and Engage in Any Order

What's great about ACT is that if you ever find yourself stuck—in life or just on a particular process in ACT—you can actually get yourself "unstuck" and more psychologically flexible by engaging with *any other ACT process*. Rigidity is the enemy of ACT and thus the enemy of your well-being. So let's take a moment to review the model and then put it all together.

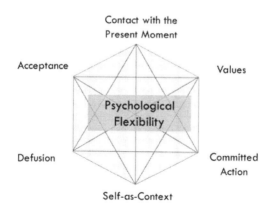

The Hexaflex Model of Psychological Flexibility
(reprinted with permission from Hayes et al, 2012)

As you can see from the diagram, the six core processes are connected and they all flow into and contribute to psychological flexibility. You can enhance each core process by not only working on that process, but by *coming at it through the other processes*. You may have noticed that there's a certain degree of overlap in the model. For example:

- Engaging in committed action requires good values work.
- Being fully present in the moment, requires some level of acceptance.
- Self-as-context is defusion applied to the self instead of individual thoughts.

The fluidity of the model means that no ACT process occurs in isolation from the other processes. They are connected to one another, not just in the diagram but in your life. So, when you get stuck—and you will get stuck, because we all do—rather than hammer away at one process, simply tap into another that you may feel more connected to at that moment. You don't always have to open up in order to engage. Sometimes you can use engagement as a way to open up. In short, if you're struggling with one process, try another. Do what works when it works. It doesn't make sense to do it any other way.

As you practice more and more you'll come to realize that working each process in isolation, while better than not working a process at all, is not as effective as working them as part of a connected whole. Because each process is connected to the others, your ability to move flexibly between them will greatly enhance your psychological flexibility. This will increase the richness and quality of your life—in good times and bad as you navigate any circumstances throughout your extraordinary lifetime.

Isolation Is the Enemy, Connection Is the Cure

In the same way you don't want to address the core processes of ACT in isolation but rather in their connectedness, you also want to be connected to others in your life. There's a mountain of scientific research that consistently highlights the impact of social relationships on our quality of life. Generally, the more connected we are (we're talking quality here, not necessarily quantity) the healthier we are—physically, emotionally, psychologically, and spiritually. The more disconnected we are, the worse we tend to fare and the harder it is to cope, especially during difficult times.

The pandemic has been an extremely challenging time and has likely affected you in a way that's not in line with who you are. You may be irritable, less interactive, less engaged, or have less energy. It takes effort to connect with people, particularly if you're not feeling well, if you're uncomfortable with your circumstances, and if you're feeling vulnerable. Other people might also be distancing themselves for similar reasons. Remember, you're not the only one who may try to avoid uncomfortable thoughts and feelings. Additionally, the burdens on you and your family could be putting a strain on these relationships making them less enjoyable and, at worst, more difficult.

All of these factors and many more can contribute to a lack of connection with people, which can take a significant toll. Additionally, reaching out for that connection may be met with a variety of responses, and some of them might be downright hurtful. None of this is anyone's fault. COVID-19 has infected the entire world, even if the virus hasn't invaded everyone's body.

However, you have the opportunity to approach your life from a place of psychological flexibility. If you're able to integrate the ACT model, it may dramatically impact these dynamics and increase the likelihood that you're able to maintain healthy relationships and even make new ones. I would encourage all of your family members or anyone close to you to read this book as well, so you can work with one another to be more flexible and stay connected as you create your future together.

The bottom line is that in the ACT model and in life, isolation is the enemy. Look for the connections and the flexibility in the model to help you better engage with it in your life, and look for the same in your relationships. You will reap the rewards in ways that might surprise you.

Julie's Connection Story

I was in England in 1995, not long after they launched the national lottery. Everyone was asking each other, "how do you pick your numbers?" I heard it in pubs, at the train station, waiting in lines, everywhere. When I saw an elderly granny ask a punk rocker with a tall pink mohawk about his numbers (they were clearly strangers), it hit me how unifying a shared experience can be.

Difficult as it's been, we have the pandemic in common with everyone in the world now. That's absolutely astonishing to me. And I'm in awe of what my friends and family have done during hard times in the midst of struggles. They've schooled their kids, delivered food, volunteered, taken care of each other, figured out new technology, kept their businesses afloat, worked in dangerous conditions, coped with unreasonable work burdens, learned new skills, moved on for the better, changed careers, finished long languishing novels, excelled in school, gotten into college, and so much more. If it's shown me anything it's that we're creative, hopeful, and resilient in the face of adversity— *extraordinary people in extraordinary times.*

As much as I love my people, I hibernate when I'm low. I don't want to be negative with my friends and family. But I challenged myself to reach out, even if only in small ways, when I was feeling awful. And, of course, the people I love bring out the best in me, so I didn't bring my worst to them at all.

After my husband hurt his knee, there were days when I was really struggling. Against my natural tendencies, I asked for help. This was extremely uncomfortable for me. Everyone I asked to help or take over a responsibility or cut me some slack was generous beyond my imagination. I was grateful and deeply touched by this. I can honestly say my relationships are as good as they've ever been. So, I'll grudgingly concede that connection beats isolation.

Julie's Tip: For me, ACT has successfully made a lifetime of unhelpful advice click—"It's not life and death" (defusion), "you can't do anything about the past" (contact with the present moment), "follow your bliss" (values/committed action). Despite my lack of success with these tips, I've passed mine on to you as if they'd be helpful. If they're not, there's a lot of great information out there. So, find what works for you because ACT works!

Chapter 10

Resetting Our Future—Starting Now

The future depends on what you do today.
—Mahatma Gandhi

Lead by Example

As this book is a part of a series about Resetting Our Future, I'd like to take a moment to directly address the subject of moving forward. I am a scientist at heart, so I rely on clinical trials and empirical evidence to see the big picture. While ACT is a scientifically solid model, the cold hard facts about its use by people who are suffering from a pandemic are lacking, naturally. However, as a psychologist, I work in the realm of individual choice, which is truly where all change takes place. So, while I can't extrapolate into the future based on evidence of any kind, I have offered my best advice for how you can move forward and make meaningful choices that could have a lasting positive impact.

If there's one truism that underlies our collective rebuilding efforts it's that we're all responsible for ourselves. You only have control over your own choices and behaviors. It's a cliché for a reason: *You have to be the change you want to see in the world.* You can take heart in knowing that even the smallest choices grounded in firm values can yield powerful positive results.

Consider the Ripple Effect

Take a moment to reflect on your own experience with the pandemic and the negative impact it's had on the people you love. Then think of all of the people you know who have also experienced pandemic-related struggles. Now picture the whole world and imagine the ripple effect. Let that sink in. However, if it's true that our behavior has an effect on others—for better or worse—it is within our ability to create a positive ripple effect.

It might seem overly optimistic to think our choices can change the world, but it's safe to say our actions have consequences that impact others:

- When you observe without judgment, you have more compassion for others.
- When you act according to your values, it is easier to see the values that underpin the actions of others, giving us more understanding and respect for their choices.
- When you act with kindness, compassion, and openness, you pass those qualities on to others.

Remember the values exercise where you were asked to think about someone you admired? If you had someone in mind and if you aimed to emulate that person, this is a perfect example of how the actions of one individual have radiated into the world in a positive way. This positive ripple effect is as real and as influential as a negative one.

There will always be people who are willing to help make the world a better place, and you may be one of them. These are certainly unprecedented times. We've never had the ability to reach out to so many friends, acquaintances, or even total strangers with a few keystrokes. But even if you don't have aspirations to change the world or reach out to strangers, you still have influence. What you do matters for yourself and the people you love. Always remember that right here and now is all you have, and it's no small feat to live a values-driven life while you stay connected to the people you love.

Only you have the ability to change. Of course, change is uncomfortable, but the pandemic has forced the issue. We've already let go of the familiar, and there's no well-worn path to return to. Simply put, we have no choice but to forge a new one.

It might be difficult to do well, but with your values and these ACT tools, you don't need a roadmap. You've got a compass, and it's guiding you on a path that is full of meaningful experiences. If you share your life and connect with others, you might also serve as an inspiration to the people you know, by being exactly who you are. And this would be extraordinary.

My Hope for You

It is my sincere hope that this book has positively impacted your life and will continue to be of some help to you. My own clinical experience tells me that ACT can be a powerful intervention. In fact, you're holding this book because I believe so strongly that all people who are suffering can benefit from it.

I can't overstate the severity of the impact the pandemic has had on the lives of so many—too many. It has been devastating. With so much loss and pain, you might feel like you're a completely different person. *You are not.* And I believe that ACT can help you reclaim your life—your very identity—from COVID-19.

In my practice, I've seen that ACT is absolutely a viable approach to leading a richer, fuller, and more meaningful life. It can protect you from being defined by the circumstances of your life. (You get to decide who you are!) Moreover, no matter what comes your way, ACT will be with you. It's more than a system for coping with hardship—it's a way to approach your life all the time, at any stage.

If anything on these pages has resonated with you, I strongly encourage you to seek out other ACT resources. There are many out there produced by people far more steeped and knowledgeable in ACT than I am. Learning more from them will be to your benefit. Also, please feel free to educate others about ACT and share your story if it's of value to you. It is, after all, our connections with one another that will help us all to rise above human suffering.

From the Authors

It is our sincere hope that you got something valuable from this book and that it lightens your burdens. If so, please recommend it to anyone you know who might be suffering and feel free to review it at your favorite online site. We wish you well and urge you again to connect with others and be compassionate with yourself. You are not alone.

Sincerely, Joseph J. Trunzo and Julie Luongo

Recommended Reading

Dahl, J., Wilson, K. G., Luciano, C., and Hayes, S. C. (2005). *Acceptance and Commitment Therapy for Chronic Pain*. Context Press: Reno, NV.

Frankl, Viktor (2006). *Man's Search for Meaning*. Beacon Press: Boston, MA.

Harris, R. (2009). *ACT Made Simple: A Quick Start Guide to ACT Basics and Beyond*. New Harbinger: Oakland, CA.

Hayes, S. C. and Smith, S. (2005). *Get Out of Your Mind and Into Your Life: The New Acceptance and Commitment Therapy*. New Harbinger: Oakland, CA.

Hayes, S. C., Strosahl, K. D., and Wilson, K. G. (2012). *Acceptance and Commitment Therapy: The Process and Practice of Mindful Change*, 2nd Ed. Guilford: New York, NY.

Hayes, S. C., Strosahl, K., and Wilson, K. G. (1999). *Acceptance and Commitment Therapy: An Experiential Approach to Behavior Change*. Guilford Press: New York, NY.

McCracken, L. M. (Ed.) (2011), *Mindfulness and Acceptance in Behavioral Medicine: Current theory and practice*. New Harbinger: Oakland, CA.

Stoddard, J. A. and Afari, N. (2014). *The Big Book of ACT Metaphors*. New Harbinger: Oakland

Trunzo, J. J. (2018). *Living Beyond Lyme: Reclaim Your Life From Lyme Disease and Chronic Illness*. Changemakers Books; United Kingdom.

Williams, J. M. G. and Kabat-Zinn, J. (2013). *Mindfulness: Diverse Perspectives on its Meaning, Origins and Applications*. Routledge: New York, NY.

Wilson, K. G. and DuFrene, T. (2010). *Things might go terribly, horribly wrong: A guide to life liberated from anxiety*. New Harbinger: Oakland, CA.

CHANGEMAKERS
BOOKS

Transform your life, transform our world. Changemakers
Books publishes books for people who seek to become positive,
powerful agents of change. These books inform, inspire, and
provide practical wisdom and skills to empower us to write
the next chapter of humanity's future.
www.changemakers-books.com

The *Resilience* Series

The Resilience Series is a collaborative effort by the authors of Changemakers Books in response to the 2020 coronavirus pandemic. Each concise volume offers expert advice and practical exercises for mastering specific skills and abilities. Our intention is that by strengthening your resilience, you can better survive and even thrive in a time of crisis.
www.resiliencebooks.com

Adapt and Plan for the New Abnormal – in the COVID-19 Coronavirus Pandemic
Gleb Tsipursky

Aging with Vision, Hope and Courage in a Time of Crisis
John C. Robinson

Connecting with Nature in a Time of Crisis
Melanie Choukas-Bradley

Going Within in a Time of Crisis
P. T. Mistlberger

Grow Stronger in a Time of Crisis
Linda Ferguson

Handling Anxiety in a Time of Crisis
George Hoffman

Navigating Loss in a Time of Crisis
Jules De Vitto

The Life-Saving Skill of Story
Michelle Auerbach

Virtual Teams – Holding the Center When You Can't Meet Face-to-Face
Carlos Valdes-Dapena

Virtually Speaking – Communicating at a Distance
Tim Ward and Teresa Erickson

Current Bestsellers from Changemakers Books

Pro Truth
A Practical Plan for Putting Truth Back into Politics
Gleb Tsipursky and Tim Ward

How can we turn back the tide of post-truth politics, fake news, and misinformation that is damaging our democracy? In the lead up to the 2020 US Presidential Election, Pro Truth provides the answers.

An Antidote to Violence
Evaluating the Evidence
Barry Spivack and Patricia Anne Saunders

It's widely accepted that Transcendental Meditation can create peace for the individual, but can it create peace in society as a whole? And if it can, what could possibly be the mechanism?

Finding Solace at Theodore Roosevelt Island
Melanie Choukas-Bradley

A woman seeks solace on an urban island paradise in Washington D.C. through 2016–17, and the shock of the Trump election.

the bottom
a theopoetic of the streets
Charles Lattimore Howard

An exploration of homelessness fusing theology, jazz-verse and intimate storytelling into a challenging, raw and beautiful tale.

The Soul of Activism
A Spirituality for Social Change
Shmuly Yanklowitz

A unique examination of the power of interfaith spirituality to fuel the fires of progressive activism.

Future Consciousness
The Path to Purposeful Evolution
Thomas Lombardo

An empowering evolutionary vision of wisdom and the human mind to guide us in creating a positive future.

Preparing for a World that Doesn't Exist – Yet
Rick Smyre and Neil Richardson

This book is about an emerging Second Enlightenment and the capacities you will need to achieve success in this new, fast-evolving world.